A - Z of Mental Health

A - Z

Andrew D Beattie

Published by Andrew D Beattie, 2023.

Table of Contents

A – Z

Of Mental Health

Written by

Andrew D Beattie

Dedicated to:

This book is dedicated to all the brave souls who wake up every day fighting battles within their own minds. To those who face the challenges that mental health issues bring—your resilience is awe-inspiring and your strength unparalleled.

I also extend this dedication to the caregivers, family members, friends, and healthcare providers who stand steadfastly beside those grappling with mental health conditions. Your support, often rendered in quiet ways, makes an immeasurable difference and illuminates the path to recovery and understanding.

May this work serve as a companion on your journey, a resource in times of uncertainty, and a testament to the collective struggle and triumph that comes with navigating the intricate landscape of mental health.

With heartfelt respect and endless hope for brighter days,

Andrew D Beattie

Introduction

Welcome to "A to Z of Mental Health," a comprehensive guide designed to demystify the complex landscape of mental well-being. Whether you have found this book out of personal necessity, academic curiosity, or the will to support someone you care about, you have come to a place where understanding meets empathy.

The realm of mental health is as vast as it is intricate. In a world that is just beginning to shed the stigmas associated with mental illness, there remains a pressing need for reliable information and compassionate dialogue. This book aims to meet that need, serving as both a resource and a companion in your journey toward understanding mental health better.

From Cluster A, B, and C personality disorders to conditions that fall outside these categories, this book offers an exhaustive list of terms, conditions, and concerns that populate the mental health field. You'll discover not just definitions, but also symptoms, treatments, and—where relevant—legal and ethical considerations, particularly focusing on the UK landscape.

But this book is more than just an encyclopedic tour. It's a call to action. It's a call to eliminate the stigma surrounding mental health, one that has persisted for far too long, isolating individuals and hindering effective treatment. The societal attitudes towards mental health are undergoing transformation, and through information and understanding, we can all be a part of this essential change.

We'll also explore the resources available to those seeking help, from global organizations to UK-specific helplines, including some based in Scotland. Every chapter aims to empower you with knowledge, so you can make well-informed choices whether you're dealing with these issues personally, professionally, or academically.

In a society that is increasingly acknowledging the importance of mental well-being alongside physical health, the need for a straightforward, inclusive, and compassionate discussion is more crucial than ever. This book is a step in that direction.

What Causes Mental Health Conditions?

The causes of mental health conditions are complex and multifaceted, often involving a combination of factors rather than a single root cause. It's essential to note that what may trigger a mental health condition in one person may not necessarily have the same impact on another. Here are some common contributing factors:

Genetic Factors

A FAMILY HISTORY OF mental health disorders can make some individuals more susceptible. However, having a family member with a mental health condition doesn't guarantee that one will develop a condition themselves.

Environmental Factors

EXTERNAL CIRCUMSTANCES such as trauma, extreme stress, abuse, and neglect can contribute to the onset of mental health conditions. Socioeconomic factors, including poverty and lack of access to quality healthcare, can also play a role.

Biological Factors

NEUROTRANSMITTER IMBALANCES, hormonal fluctuations, and other physiological factors can contribute to mental health issues. Some medical conditions, like thyroid disorders, can also produce symptoms resembling mental health conditions.

Psychological Factors

LONG-STANDING PATTERNS of negative thinking, poor self-esteem, and maladaptive coping mechanisms can contribute to mental health conditions. Personal experiences like early childhood trauma or being part of a marginalized community can also be factors.

Lifestyle Choices

SUBSTANCE ABUSE, INCLUDING excessive alcohol consumption and drug misuse, can lead to mental health issues or exacerbate existing ones. Lack of physical activity and poor diet can also contribute.

Cultural Factors

STIGMA, DISCRIMINATION, and culturally induced stress can also play a role, especially in communities where mental health issues are not well understood or are stigmatized.

Co-morbidity

THE PRESENCE OF ONE mental health condition can sometimes contribute to the development of another, complicating both diagnosis and treatment.

It's usually a mix of these factors that leads to mental health conditions, and identifying the specific causes can be a complicated process that involves thorough assessment, including medical tests, psychological evaluations, and history-taking. Treatment is often similarly multi-pronged, addressing both the symptoms and the underlying contributing factors.

PART I: Why You Need an A-Z of Mental Health Definitions

Mental health is a complex and diverse topic that affects millions of people around the world. However, many people lack the knowledge and understanding of the various terms and concepts related to mental health. This can lead to confusion, stigma, discrimination, and barriers to seeking help.

That's why having an A-Z of mental health definitions can be very useful and beneficial for anyone who wants to learn more about this important subject. An A-Z of mental health definitions is a comprehensive and accessible guide that provides clear and concise explanations of the most common and relevant terms and concepts in mental health.

By reading this book, you will be able to:

- Gain a better understanding of your own mental health and well-being, as well as the mental health of others.
- Recognize the signs and symptoms of different mental health conditions and disorders and know when to seek professional help.
- Learn about the causes, risk factors, prevention, and treatment options for various mental health issues.
- Discover the latest research and developments in the field of mental health.

- Reduce the stigma and misconceptions that surround mental health and promote a more positive and supportive attitude towards it.

Whether you are a student, a professional, a caregiver, or simply someone who is curious and interested in mental health, this book will provide you with valuable information and insights that will enhance your knowledge and awareness of this vital topic. You will also find helpful resources and references for further reading and exploration.

Chapter 1: A is for Apple

———

It is also for:

1. **ADHD stands for Attention-Deficit/ Hyperactivity Disorder.** It is a neurodevelopmental disorder characterized by persistent patterns of inattention, impulsivity, and/or hyperactivity. These symptoms can interfere with daily functioning and quality of life. ADHD is commonly diagnosed in childhood but can persist into adulthood. Treatment often involves a combination of medication, behavioral therapy, and lifestyle changes.

2. **Agoraphobia** - A type of anxiety disorder characterized by extreme fear of places or situations that might cause panic, helplessness, or embarrassment, often leading to avoidance behaviour.

3. **Anorexia Nervosa** - An eating disorder marked by an intense fear of gaining weight and a distorted body image, resulting in self-imposed starvation and excessive weight loss.

4. **Anxiety Disorder** - A general term for disorders characterized by excessive fear, anxiety, or avoidance behaviour, which may include generalized anxiety disorder, panic disorder, and social anxiety disorder among others.

5. **Antisocial Personality Disorder** - A personality disorder characterized by a persistent pattern of

disregard for the rights of others and lack of empathy.

6. **Asperger's Syndrome** - Part of the Autism Spectrum Disorder, it's characterized by difficulties in social interaction and nonverbal communication, along with restricted interests and repetitive behaviours. Note that the term is being used less frequently in favour of Autism Spectrum Disorder.

7. **Attachment Disorder** - A broad term describing disorders of mood, behaviour, and social relationships arising from a failure to form normal attachments to primary caregivers in early childhood.

8. **Atypical Depression** - A subtype of depression that includes mood reactivity, increased appetite or weight gain, excessive sleep, and sensitivity to rejection.

9. **Autistic Spectrum Disorder (ASD)** - A developmental disorder characterized by difficulties with social interaction and communication, along with restricted interests and repetitive behaviours.

10. **Avoidant Personality Disorder** - A personality disorder characterized by extreme shyness, feelings of inadequacy, and a fear of rejection, leading to avoidance of social interactions and relationships.

11. **Adjustment Disorder** - A short-term emotional or behavioural reaction to a stressful event or change in a person's life, which is considered maladaptive or somehow not an expected healthy response to the event or change.

These are general definitions, and the manifestations of these conditions can vary widely from person to person.

Chapter 2: B is for....

1. **Bipolar Disorder** - A mental health condition characterized by extreme mood swings that include emotional highs (mania or hypomania) and lows (depression).
2. **Borderline Personality Disorder (BPD)** - A mental health disorder characterized by unstable moods, behaviour, and relationships, often with intense emotional reactions and impulsivity.
3. **Body Dysmorphic Disorder (BDD)** - A psychological disorder in which a person becomes obsessed with imagined defects in their physical appearance.
4. **Bulimia Nervosa** - An eating disorder characterized by episodes of binge eating followed by behaviours to prevent weight gain, such as vomiting, excessive exercise, or laxative use.
5. **Brief Psychotic Disorder** - A mental condition characterized by a short-term episode of psychotic symptoms such as hallucinations and delusions.
6. **Bereavement** - The psychological process of coping with a loss, usually referring to grief, which is a normal reaction to the death of a loved one.
7. **Behavioural Addiction** - A form of addiction that involves a compulsion to engage in a rewarding non-substance-related behaviour, such as gambling, despite negative consequences.

8. **Brooding** - A mental state characterized by persistent, obsessive, and often negative thinking.

9. **Burnout** - A state of emotional, mental, and often physical exhaustion brought on by prolonged or repeated stress, usually in a work context.

10. **Body Integrity Dysphoria (or Body Integrity Identity Disorder)** - A psychological disorder in which an individual experiences a strong desire to amputate a healthy limb or has the desire for some other form of disability.

These definitions provide a general overview, and the symptoms and experiences can vary from individual to individual.

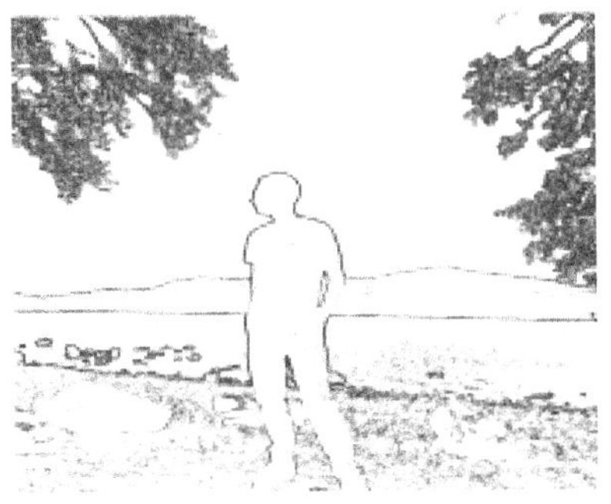

Chapter 3: C is for ....

1. **Cognitive Behavioural Therapy (CBT)** - A type of psychotherapy that focuses on identifying and challenging distorted thought patterns and beliefs to improve emotional regulation and coping skills.
2. **Conversion Disorder** - A psychological disorder where physical symptoms, such as paralysis or blindness, manifest without a known medical cause, often as a response to stress or trauma.
3. **Cyclothymia** - A milder form of bipolar disorder characterized by mood swings between mild depression and hypomania.
4. **Claustrophobia** - An anxiety disorder characterized by an intense fear of small or enclosed spaces.
5. **Chronic Stress** - A prolonged and constant feeling of stress that can negatively affect health.
6. **Conduct Disorder** - A behavioural and emotional disorder in children and adolescents characterized by a long-term pattern of violating the basic rights of others or societal norms.
7. **Compulsive Behaviour** - A psychological condition where an individual performs certain behaviours repeatedly, even if they wish to stop or the actions have negative consequences.
8. **Co-occurring Disorders** - The simultaneous presence of both a mental health disorder and a substance use disorder.

9. **Coprolalia** - An involuntary utterance of socially inappropriate or taboo words or phrases, often associated with Tourette's syndrome.

10. **Complex PTSD (C-PTSD)** - A form of post-traumatic stress disorder that arises from prolonged exposure to traumatic events, often including emotional abuse or neglect.

11. **Catatonia** - A behavioural syndrome marked by an inability to move normally, often seen in some psychiatric conditions like schizophrenia.

12. **Cognitive Dissonance -** The mental discomfort experienced by a person who holds two or more contradictory beliefs, values, or perceptions at the same time.

These definitions are general overviews and the symptoms and experiences of these conditions can vary from person to person.

Chapter 4: D is for...

1. **Depression** - A mood disorder characterized by persistent feelings of sadness, hopelessness, and a lack of interest or pleasure in activities.
2. **Dissociative Identity Disorder (DID)** - A severe form of dissociation involving a person experiencing two or more distinct identities or personality states, each with its own pattern of perceiving and interacting with the world.
3. **Dysthymia** - A chronic form of depression with symptoms that are less severe than major depressive disorder but last longer, often for years.
4. **Delusion** - A false belief that is resistant to reasoning or confrontation with actual facts, often found in disorders like schizophrenia.
5. **Double Depression** - A condition where persistent depressive disorder (dysthymia) and major depressive disorder occur simultaneously.
6. **Dopamine** - A neurotransmitter involved in regulating mood and emotional responses, often discussed in the context of mental health disorders like depression and schizophrenia.
7. **Depersonalization** - A form of dissociation involving a feeling of being detached from oneself or one's own body or mental processes.
8. **Derealization** - A form of dissociation where the external world feels unreal or distorted.

9. **Delirium** - A sudden and severe change in brain function that can cause confusion, hallucinations, and emotional disturbances, often due to a medical condition or substance intoxication.

10. **Disinhibition** - A lack of restraint or inability to control one's impulses, sometimes related to conditions like ADHD or frontal lobe damage.

11. **Diagnostic and Statistical Manual of Mental Disorders (DSM)** - The standard classification manual used by mental health professionals to diagnose mental disorders.

12. **Drug-Induced Psychosis** - A condition where psychotic symptoms are triggered by substance abuse or withdrawal.

These are general definitions, and the symptoms and experiences of these conditions can differ among individuals.

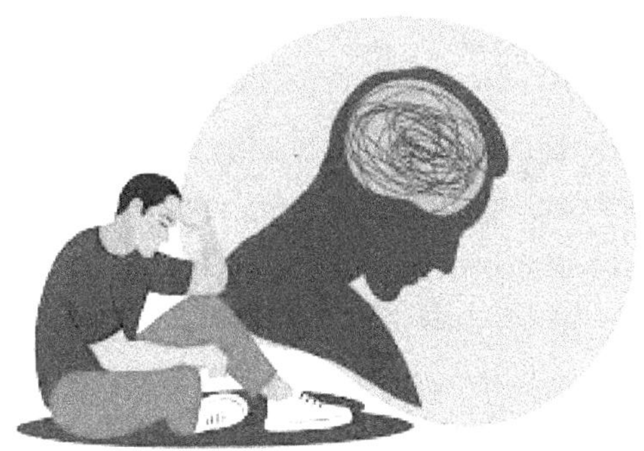

Chapter 5: E is for....

1. **Eating Disorders** - A category of mental health disorders characterized by preoccupation with food, body weight, and shape, leading to dangerous and unhealthy eating behaviours. Examples include anorexia nervosa, bulimia nervosa, and binge-eating disorder.
2. **Emotional Dysregulation** - The inability to manage emotional responses, often seen in conditions like borderline personality disorder and some mood disorders.
3. **EMDR (Eye Movement Desensitization and Reprocessing)** - A psychotherapy technique used to help individuals process traumatic memories.
4. **Emotional Intelligence** - The ability to recognize, understand, and manage one's own emotions, as well as to recognize, understand, and influence the emotions of others.
5. **Executive Function** - A set of mental skills that help with managing time, paying attention, changing focus, planning, organizing, and remembering details. Deficits in executive function are often seen in conditions like ADHD.
6. **Exposure Therapy** - A psychological treatment that helps individuals confront their fears and anxieties by gradually and systematically exposing them to the feared object or situation.

7. **Enabling** - A pattern of behaviour often seen in relationships with substance abusers, where a person inadvertently helps sustain the individual's addiction.

8. **Electroconvulsive Therapy (ECT)** - A medical procedure used in the treatment of severe depression and other mental illnesses, where electrical currents are passed through the brain to trigger a seizure.

9. **Erotomania** - A delusional belief that a specific person, often a celebrity or someone in a position of authority, is in love with the individual.

10. **Existential Crisis** - A moment when an individual questions the very foundations of their life, often related to concerns about the meaning, purpose, or value of life.

11. **Emotional Abuse** - A form of abuse that involves the manipulation and degradation of the victim's emotional well-being, often through verbal abuse or excessive control.

12. **Euthymia** - A term often used to describe a stable, relatively balanced mood state, which is neither highly elated nor severely depressed.

These are general definitions, and symptoms or experiences can differ from person to person

Chapter 6: F is for ......

1. **Freudian Psychology** - A school of psychology founded by Sigmund Freud that focuses on unconscious drives and the role of early experiences in shaping personality and mental health.
2. **Flooding** - A type of exposure therapy where a person is rapidly and intensely exposed to their fear-provoking stimuli, usually in a controlled setting.
3. **Flight-or-Fight Response** - A physiological reaction that occurs in response to a perceived harmful event, attack, or threat, often discussed in the context of anxiety and stress disorders.
4. **Free Association** - A psychoanalytic technique in which patients are encouraged to share thoughts, words, or images that come to mind, often used to uncover underlying issues.
5. **Frontal Lobe** - A region of the brain associated with higher cognitive functions like planning, reasoning, and self-control; its dysfunction can contribute to various mental health disorders.
6. **Factitious Disorder** - A mental health condition in which a person acts as if they have an illness by deliberately producing or faking symptoms.
7. **Fugue State** - A rare psychiatric disorder characterized by reversible amnesia for personal identity, often involving unplanned travel or wandering.

8. **Family Therapy** - A type of psychological counselling that aims to improve communication and resolve conflicts within a family, often used for treating conditions like eating disorders, substance abuse, and mood disorders.

9. **Functional MRI (fMRI)** - A neuroimaging technique used to observe brain activity, often used in research on mental health conditions.

10. **Formication** - The sensation of insects crawling on or under the skin, sometimes a symptom of substance abuse or certain mental health conditions.

11. **Folie à Deux** - A psychiatric syndrome in which symptoms of a delusional belief are shared among two or more individuals.

12. **Flat Affect** - A lack of emotional expression, often seen in conditions like schizophrenia or severe depression.

These definitions are intended to provide a general overview, and the symptoms and experiences can differ among individuals.

Chapter 7: G is for...

1. **Generalized Anxiety Disorder (GAD)** - A chronic anxiety disorder characterized by excessive, long-lasting worry and fear about everyday situations.
2. **Group Therapy** - A form of psychotherapy where multiple patients meet to describe and discuss their problems together, facilitated by a therapist.
3. **Grandiosity** - An exaggerated sense of one's own importance or abilities, often seen in conditions like narcissistic personality disorder or manic phases of bipolar disorder.
4. **Gestalt Therapy** - A form of psychotherapy that focuses on an individual's present experience, perception, and functioning in the context of their environment.
5. **Grey Matter** - Brain tissue consisting mainly of cell bodies and branching dendrites, often discussed in the context of mental health research.
6. **Gender Dysphoria** - Psychological distress stemming from a discrepancy between a person's gender identity and their assigned sex at birth.
7. **Grief Counselling** - A form of psychotherapy aimed at helping individuals cope with the emotional and mental stress after the loss of a loved one.
8. **General Adaptation Syndrome** - A model describing the body's short-term and long-term reactions to stress, often cited in discussions of

anxiety and stress disorders.

9. **Genetic Predisposition** - The increased likelihood of developing a particular disease or condition based on one's genetic makeup, often discussed in the context of mental health disorders.

10. **Guilt** - A complex emotion that occurs when a person believes they have done something wrong, often discussed in the context of depression or anxiety disorders.

11. **Gaslighting** - A form of emotional abuse involving the manipulation of someone into doubting their own reality or perceptions.

12. **Graphomania** - An obsessive impulse to write, often related to a manic state in bipolar disorder.

These definitions are general overviews, and symptoms or experiences can differ from person to person.

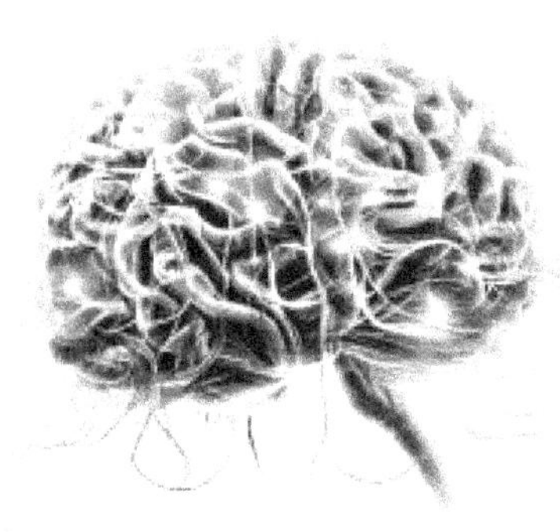

Chapter 8: H is for...

1. **Hypomania** - A milder form of mania characterized by elevated mood and increased activity, often seen in bipolar disorder.
2. **Hallucination** - A perception of something that is not present in the external environment, commonly associated with conditions like schizophrenia.
3. **Hoarding Disorder** - A mental health disorder characterized by persistent difficulty discarding possessions, leading to clutter and distress.
4. **Histrionic Personality Disorder** - A personality disorder marked by excessive attention-seeking behaviour and emotional instability.
5. **Habituation** - A psychological learning process wherein the response to a stimulus decreases after repeated exposure, often discussed in the context of therapy for phobias or anxiety.
6. **Hypochondria (now often called Illness Anxiety Disorder)** - Excessive preoccupation or worry about having a serious illness, despite having little or no medical evidence to support the presence of an illness.
7. **Hyperactivity** - An elevated level of activity that may be goal-directed or aimless, often associated with conditions like ADHD.
8. **Hypnosis** - A therapeutic technique intended to induce a state of increased receptivity to suggestion

and altered consciousness, used in some mental health treatments.

9. **Harm Reduction** - Strategies and techniques aimed at reducing the negative consequences associated with certain behaviours, such as substance abuse.

10. **Hyperarousal** - A heightened state of sensory sensitivity accompanied by an exaggerated intensity of behaviours, often seen in conditions like PTSD.

11. **Humanistic Psychology** - A psychological perspective emphasizing individual growth, free will, and the importance of subjective experience.

12. **Health Anxiety** - Excessive worrying about one's health, often to the point where it interferes with daily life, sometimes referred to as Illness Anxiety Disorder.

These definitions provide a general overview, and symptoms or experiences can differ from person to person.

Chapter 9: I is for...

1. **Insomnia** - Difficulty falling asleep or staying asleep, often associated with various mental health conditions like anxiety and depression.
2. **Impulse Control Disorders** - A class of psychiatric disorders characterized by the inability to resist urges or impulses, leading to potentially harmful behaviour.
3. **Intermittent Explosive Disorder** - A disorder characterized by sudden episodes of unwarranted anger or aggression, usually lasting less than 30 minutes.
4. **Irritable Bowel Syndrome (IBS)** - A gastrointestinal disorder often linked with stress and mental health issues like anxiety and depression.
5. **Imagery Rehearsal Therapy** - A cognitive-behavioural therapy used to treat nightmares and night terrors, often related to PTSD.
6. **Intellectual Disability** - A disorder marked by significant limitations in both intellectual functioning and adaptive behaviour, originating before the age of 18.
7. **Informed Consent** - The ethical and legal requirement for a healthcare provider to explain the risks, benefits, and alternatives of a treatment to a patient.
8. **Introversion** - A personality trait characterized by a preference for solitary activities over social

interaction, not necessarily linked to a mental health condition but often discussed in psychological literature.

9. **Isolation** - The experience of being separated from others, which can be both a symptom and a contributing factor for various mental health issues.
10. **Id** - In Freudian psychology, the part of the mind that is driven by basic urges and desires.
11. **Inattention** - A lack of focus or concentration, often associated with disorders like ADHD.
12. **Illness Anxiety Disorder** - Previously known as hypochondria, it's characterized by excessive worry about having a serious illness despite having no or only mild symptoms.

These definitions are general overviews, and symptoms or experiences can differ from person to person.

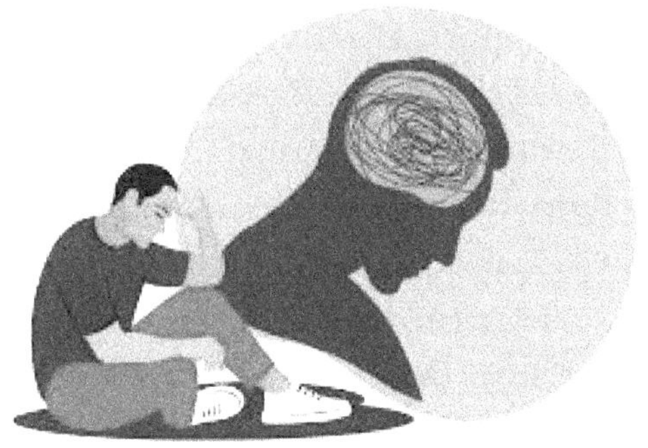

Chapter 10: J is for...

1. **Jungian Psychology** - A school of psychology founded by Carl Jung that emphasizes the role of the unconscious and archetypes in human behaviour and mental health.
2. **Jealousy** - An emotional state that may involve feelings of insecurity, fear, or envy, often discussed in the context of relationship issues or personality disorders.
3. **Journal Therapy** - A therapeutic technique that involves writing down thoughts, feelings, and experiences as a form of self-exploration and emotional processing.
4. **Judgement** - The cognitive ability to assess situations and draw appropriate conclusions; impairments are often seen in various mental disorders.
5. **Juvenile Bipolar Disorder** - The diagnosis of bipolar disorder in children or adolescents, characterized by mood swings between mania and depression.
6. **Job Burnout** - A state of emotional, physical, and mental exhaustion caused by excessive and prolonged stress, often related to work.
7. **James-Lange Theory** - A psychological theory that suggests that emotional experience is a reaction to bodily changes that occur as a result of an external situation.
8. **Just-World Hypothesis** - A cognitive bias wherein

people believe that the world is fair and that individuals get what they deserve, often discussed in the context of victim-blaming.

9. **Jargon Aphasia** - A type of language disorder common in certain types of brain damage, where speech is filled with unknown or irrelevant words.

10. **Jumping to Conclusions** - A cognitive distortion involving making quick assumptions without sufficient evidence, often seen in anxiety and other mood disorders.

11. **Juvenile Delinquency** - Illegal or antisocial behaviour in children or adolescents, sometimes associated with conduct disorder or other mental health conditions.

12. **Joining** - A therapy technique where the therapist aligns with the client's experiences to build rapport and facilitate treatment.

These definitions are general overviews, and symptoms or experiences can differ from person to person.

Chapter 11: K is for...

1. **Kleptomania** - An impulse control disorder characterized by the recurrent urge to steal items, usually without need or monetary value.
2. **Kinesthetic** - Relating to the sense of bodily movement, often discussed in the context of sensory processing issues, or learning styles.
3. **Kohlberg's Stages of Moral Development** - A psychological theory outlining how moral reasoning develops in individuals, often used in developmental psychology.
4. **Korsakoff's Syndrome** - A chronic memory disorder, usually caused by severe thiamine (vitamin B-1) deficiency, often associated with alcohol abuse.
5. **Kinesics** - The study of body language and gestures, particularly as they influence communication.
6. **Key Informant** - A person who provides specialized information or insight, often used in psychological or sociological research.
7. **Ketamine Therapy** - The clinical use of ketamine, a dissociative anaesthetic, for treating conditions like severe depression.
8. **Kindling** - A neurological phenomenon where repeated exposure to sub-threshold stimuli can lead to an exaggerated response, often discussed in relation to mood disorders.
9. **Kundalini** - A concept from Eastern philosophy

referring to a form of primal energy or life force; sometimes discussed in the context of mental health and well-being.

10. **Knowledge Deficit** - A lack of essential information, often seen in conditions like learning disabilities or in situations where patient education is needed for treatment compliance.

These definitions are general overviews, and symptoms or experiences can differ from person to person.

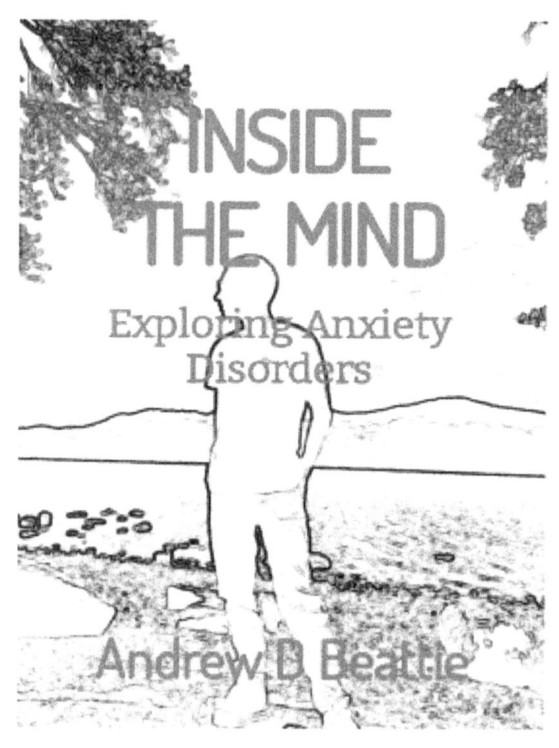
INSIDE
THE MIND
Exploring Anxiety
Disorders
Andrew D Beattie

Chapter 12: L is for...

———

1. **Learning Disability** - A neurological disorder that affects the ability to receive, process, store, or respond to information, impacting academic performance.
2. **Limbic System** - A complex system of nerves and networks in the brain, involved in emotions such as fear, pleasure, and anger.
3. **Logotherapy** - A type of psychotherapy that focuses on the human capacity for finding meaning in one's life, developed by Viktor Frankl.
4. **Latent Content** - In Freudian psychology, the hidden psychological meaning of a dream, as opposed to its literal content.
5. **Longitudinal Study** - A research design that follows subjects over a long period of time to observe long-term effects and changes.
6. **Lexapro** - A brand name for escitalopram, an antidepressant medication used to treat depression and generalized anxiety disorder.
7. **Lithium** - A mood stabilizer often used to treat bipolar disorder.
8. **Lethargy** - A state of tiredness, weariness, or lack of energy, often seen as a symptom in various mental health conditions.
9. **Learned Helplessness** - A mental state in which an individual believes that they cannot control or change a situation, often leading to decreased

motivation and depressive symptoms.

10. **Libido** - The energy of the sexual drive as a
    component of the life instinct, often discussed in
    psychoanalytic literature.

11. **Locus of Control** - The degree to which people
    believe that they have control over the outcome of
    events in their lives, as opposed to external forces
    having control.

12. **Life Review** - A form of reminiscence or reflective
    reviewing of one's life, often used therapeutically with
    older adults to enhance psychological well-being.

These definitions are general overviews, and symptoms or experiences can differ from person to person.

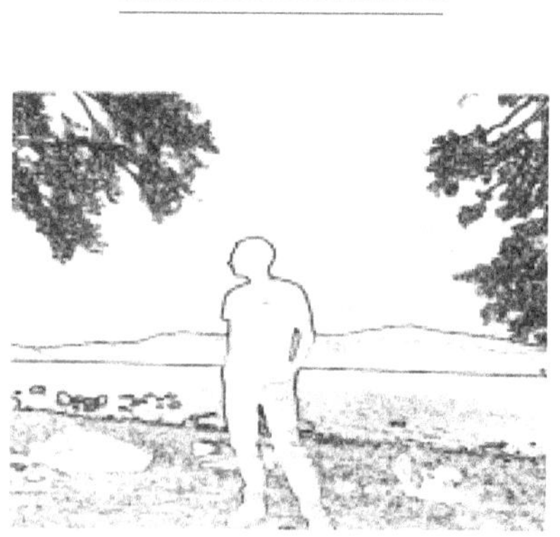

Chapter 13: M is for...

1. **Major Depressive Disorder** - A mood disorder characterized by persistent feelings of sadness, hopelessness, and a lack of interest in activities.
2. **Mania** - An elevated mood state that can include increased energy, restlessness, and sometimes impaired judgment, often seen in bipolar disorder.
3. **Mindfulness** - A therapeutic technique that involves focusing on the present moment, often used in treating anxiety and depression.
4. **Mood Stabilizers** - Medications used to treat mood swings in conditions like bipolar disorder.
5. **Maslow's Hierarchy of Needs** - A psychological theory that arranges human needs in a pyramid, with basic needs at the bottom and self-actualization at the top.
6. **Maladaptive** - Behaviours or thought patterns that are harmful or counterproductive, often discussed in the context of coping mechanisms.
7. **Malingering** - Deliberately feigning or exaggerating symptoms of a mental or physical disorder for personal gain.
8. **Melancholia** - A severe form of depression characterized by despondency, lack of interest in life, and thoughts of death or suicide.
9. **Mentalization** - The ability to understand the mental state of oneself and others, often discussed in the

context of borderline personality disorder.

10. **Multiple Personality Disorder** - An outdated term now generally referred to as Dissociative Identity Disorder, characterized by the presence of two or more distinct personality states.

11. **Myalgic Encephalomyelitis** - Also known as Chronic Fatigue Syndrome, a condition characterized by persistent, unexplained fatigue that can impact mental health.

12. **Mind-Body Connection** - The relationship between mental and physical health, suggesting that emotional or psychological stress can manifest as physical symptoms.

These definitions are general overviews, and symptoms or experiences can differ from person to person.

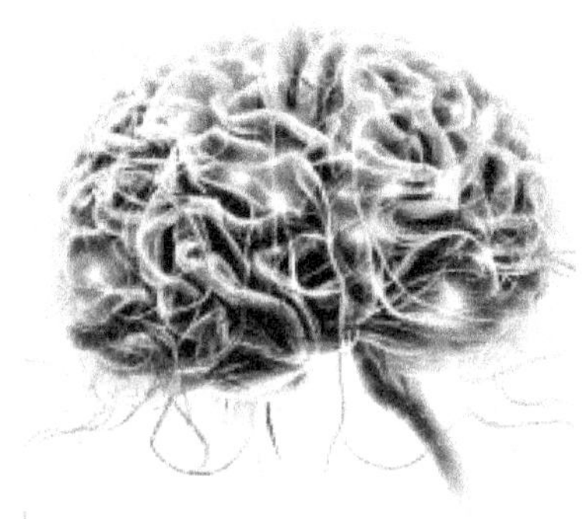

Chapter 14: N is for...

1. **Narcissistic Personality Disorder** - A mental disorder characterized by a long-term pattern of exaggerated self-importance and a lack of empathy toward others.
2. **Neurosis** - An outdated term for a range of psychological conditions characterized by high levels of anxiety or inner conflict, now often referred to as anxiety disorders.
3. **Negative Reinforcement** - A behavioural concept where the removal of an unpleasant stimulus strengthens a behaviour.
4. **Neuroplasticity** - The ability of neural networks in the brain to change through growth and reorganization, often discussed in rehabilitation and therapy contexts.
5. **Neuropsychology** - The study of the relationship between the brain and behaviour, often involved in the diagnosis and treatment of brain injuries or developmental disorders.
6. **Norepinephrine** - A neurotransmitter involved in mood regulation, attention, and the body's stress response.
7. **Non-Verbal Learning Disability** - A neurological disorder that affects the ability to interpret nonverbal cues like facial expressions and body language.
8. **Night Terrors** - Episodes of intense fear and

screaming that occur during deep sleep, often found in children and some adults.

9. **Nihilism** - A belief that life lacks purpose or value, often associated with severe depression or existential crisis.
10. **Nomophobia** - The fear of being without a mobile phone or losing mobile phone connectivity, often cited as a modern form of anxiety.
11. **Norms** - Social or cultural rules that govern behaviour, often discussed in the context of social anxiety or cultural adaptation issues.
12. **Nurturance** - Providing care, encouragement, and support, often discussed in the context of attachment theory and emotional well-being.

These definitions provide a general overview, and symptoms or experiences can differ from person to person.

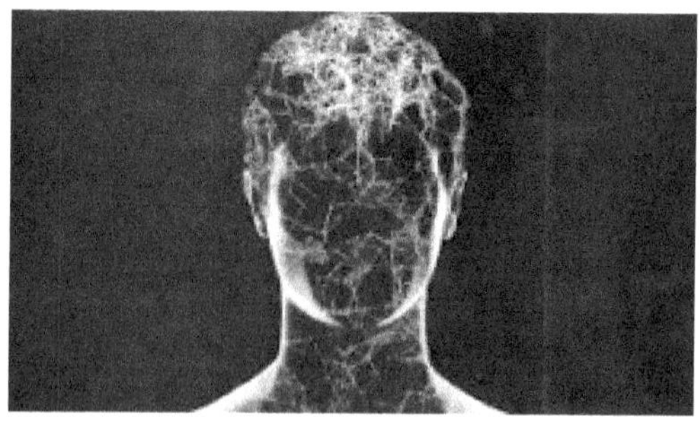

Chapter 15: O is for...

1. **Obsessive-Compulsive Disorder (OCD)** - A mental health disorder characterized by persistent, intrusive thoughts (obsessions) and repetitive behaviours or mental acts (compulsions).
2. **Oppositional Defiant Disorder (ODD)** - A childhood disorder marked by defiant, disobedient, and hostile behaviour toward authority figures.
3. **Operant Conditioning** - A type of learning in which behaviour is strengthened or weakened by the consequences that follow it.
4. **Overgeneralization** - A cognitive distortion where an individual applies the outcome of one event to all similar events, often seen in anxiety and depression.
5. **Object Relations** - A psychoanalytic concept that describes the way people relate to others based on their early experiences with caregivers.
6. **Opioid Use Disorder** - A medical condition characterized by a problematic pattern of opioid use leading to impairment or distress.
7. **Orthorexia** - An obsession with eating foods that are considered healthy, to the point where it becomes damaging to well-being.
8. **Open Dialogue** - A form of psychotherapy that involves the patient and their social network in treatment decisions and discussions.
9. **Oxytocin** - A hormone that plays a role in social

bonding, sexual reproduction, and during and after childbirth; sometimes called the "love hormone."

10. **Oneirophrenia** - A hallucinatory, dream-like state caused by various medical conditions or drug misuse.

11. **Overcompensation** - A psychological defence mechanism in which people try to cover up their weaknesses by focusing excessively on their strengths.

12. **Onychophagia** - The act of biting one's nails, often considered a sign of emotional stress, anxiety, or nervousness.

These definitions are general overviews, and symptoms or experiences can differ from person to person.

Chapter 16: P is for...

1. **Post-Traumatic Stress Disorder (PTSD)** - A mental health condition triggered by experiencing or witnessing a terrifying event, characterized by flashbacks, nightmares, and severe anxiety.
2. **Panic Disorder** - A mental health disorder characterized by recurrent panic attacks and constant fear of having future attacks.
3. **Psychotherapy** - The treatment of mental disorders through talking and psychological techniques rather than medication.
4. **Projection** - A defence mechanism where an individual attributes their own undesirable thoughts, feelings, or motives to another person.
5. **Psychosis** - A severe mental disorder characterized by a disconnection from reality, which may include hallucinations or delusions.
6. **Personality Disorder** - A class of mental disorders characterized by enduring patterns of behaviour, cognition, and inner experience, which deviate markedly from the expectations of the individual's culture.
7. **Psychopharmacology** - The study of the effects of drugs on mood, sensation, thinking, and behaviour.
8. **Placebo Effect** - The phenomenon where a patient experiences a perceived improvement due to believing they are receiving treatment, even if the

treatment has no therapeutic effect.

9. **Psychodynamic Therapy** - A form of therapy aimed at exploring unconscious thought patterns and how they influence behaviour.

10. **Positive Reinforcement** - A concept in behavioural psychology where a positive stimulus is added to encourage a behaviour.

11. **Paranoia** - A thought process characterized by excessive fear or suspicion, often seen in various mental health disorders.

12. **Psychomotor Agitation** - A series of unintentional and purposeless motions that stem from mental tension and anxiety.

These definitions are general overviews, and symptoms or experiences can differ from person to person.

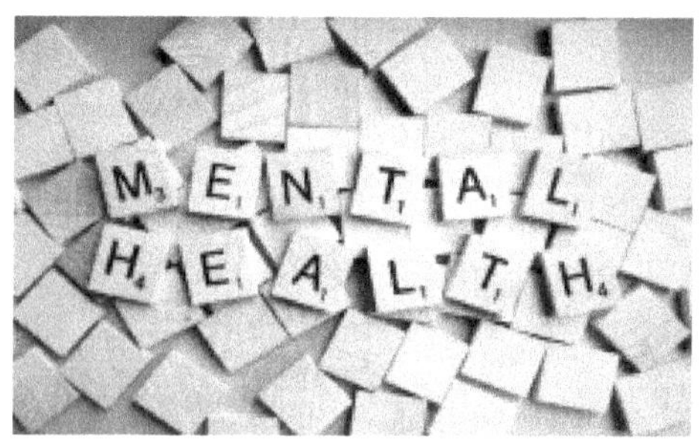

Chapter 17: Q is for...

1. **Quality of Life** - A broad concept that includes various factors like emotional well-being, physical health, and environmental conditions, often assessed in mental health studies.
2. **Quantitative Research** - Research that deals with numbers and statistical analysis, commonly used in studies related to mental health outcomes.
3. **Quetiapine** - An antipsychotic medication used to treat conditions like schizophrenia, bipolar disorder, and depression.
4. **Quiet Borderline** - A term used to describe a subtype of Borderline Personality Disorder where symptoms are primarily directed inward, rather than towards others.
5. **Quick Inventory of Depressive Symptomatology (QIDS)** - A questionnaire used to assess the severity of depressive symptoms in individuals.
6. **Quasi-Experimental Design** - A research design that lacks the full control of a true experimental design but is used to establish causal relationships, often used in mental health research.
7. **Queer Theory** - An academic field that explores sexual orientation, gender identity, and gender expression, often touching on mental health issues within the LGBTQ+ community.
8. **Questionnaire** - A set of questions used for gathering

information, commonly employed in psychological assessments and research.

9. **Qualitative Research** - Research that deals with descriptions and observations, often used to explore the intricacies of mental health conditions in a more nuanced manner.

10. **Quasi-Drug** - In some jurisdictions, a term for substances that are not classified as pharmaceuticals but are considered to have mild effects on the body, sometimes relevant in discussions about mental health supplements or alternative treatments.

These definitions provide a general overview, and symptoms or experiences can differ from person to person.

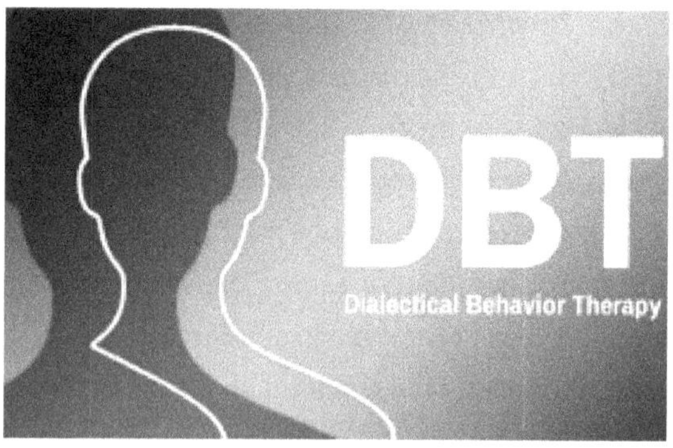

Chapter 18: R is for...

1. **Regression** - A defence mechanism where an individual reverts to an earlier stage of development in response to stress or conflict.
2. **Reinforcement** - A concept in behaviourism where a stimulus strengthens or weakens a particular behaviour.
3. **Rumination** - The act of obsessively thinking about the same thoughts or problems, often seen in conditions like depression and anxiety.
4. **Resilience** - The ability to adapt and recover quickly from adversity or stress.
5. **Repression** - A defence mechanism in which distressing memories or feelings are pushed into the unconscious mind.
6. **Recovery** - The process of overcoming a mental illness or emotional distress, often through a combination of treatment methods.
7. **Risperidone** - An antipsychotic medication used to treat conditions like schizophrenia, bipolar disorder, and irritability associated with autistic disorder.
8. **Reaction Formation** - A defence mechanism where an individual expresses the opposite of their inner feelings in order to protect themselves from the anxiety these feelings produce.
9. **Reuptake Inhibitors** - A class of drugs, such as SSRIs or SNRIs, that prevent the reabsorption of

neurotransmitters like serotonin, often used in treating depression and anxiety.

10. **Role Confusion** - A state of uncertainty or inconsistency concerning one's role in life, often discussed in the context of identity development.

11. **Repetitive Transcranial Magnetic Stimulation (rTMS)** - A non-invasive procedure that uses magnetic fields to stimulate nerve cells in the brain, used for treating depression.

12. **Rational Emotive Behaviour Therapy (REBT)** - A form of cognitive behavioural therapy that aims to help people understand the thoughts and beliefs that lead to emotional distress.

These definitions are general overviews, and symptoms or experiences can differ from person to person.

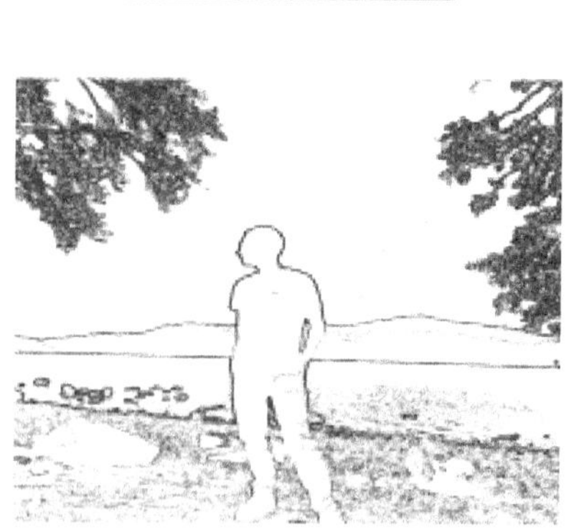

Chapter 19: S is for...

1. **Schizophrenia** - A chronic mental disorder characterized by distorted thinking, hallucinations, and a disconnection from reality.
2. **Social Anxiety Disorder** - A mental health condition marked by an intense fear of social situations, leading to avoidance and feelings of self-consciousness.
3. **Somatic Symptom Disorder** - A mental health disorder where a person experiences physical symptoms with no medical explanation, often influenced by psychological factors.
4. **Suicidal Ideation** - Thoughts of ending one's own life, ranging from fleeting considerations to detailed plans.
5. **Serotonin** - A neurotransmitter that plays a key role in mood regulation, among other functions.
6. **Substance Use Disorder** - A medical condition characterized by an inability to stop using a substance despite harmful consequences.
7. **Stigma** - A set of negative and unfair beliefs that a society has about something, often discussed in the context of mental health.
8. **Stockholm Syndrome** - A psychological phenomenon where hostages or victims develop empathy and loyalty towards their captors.
9. **Self-Esteem** - An individual's overall sense of self-

worth or value.

10. **Schema** - A mental framework that helps individuals organize and interpret information, often discussed in cognitive therapy.

11. **Selective Serotonin Reuptake Inhibitors (SSRIs)** - A class of drugs commonly used to treat depression by increasing levels of serotonin in the brain.

12. **Seasonal Affective Disorder (SAD)** - A type of depression that occurs at a specific time of year, usually in the winter when there is less natural sunlight.

These definitions are general overviews, and symptoms or experiences can differ from person to person.

Chapter 20: T is for...

1. **Trauma** - A psychological, emotional response to an event or experience that is deeply distressing or disturbing.
2. **Therapy** - The treatment of mental or psychological disorders through methods other than medication, usually involving conversation and behavioural techniques.
3. **Transference** - A psychological phenomenon where the feelings or attitudes originally associated with important figures in one's early life are unconsciously transferred to others, especially therapists.
4. **Tardive Dyskinesia** - A side effect of antipsychotic medications characterized by involuntary, repetitive body movements.
5. **Trichotillomania** - A disorder characterized by the compulsive urge to pull out one's own hair, often resulting in noticeable hair loss.
6. **Trigger** - Something that causes a negative emotional response, often used in the context of post-traumatic stress disorder or other mental health conditions.
7. **Tourette's Syndrome** - A neurological disorder characterized by repetitive, involuntary movements and vocalizations known as tics.
8. **Thought Disorder** - A mental disorder characterized by disorganized thinking, impaired reasoning, and a reduced ability to focus.

9. **Twin Studies** - Research studies that compare twins to study the relative influences of genetics and environment, often in the context of mental health.
10. **Thematic Apperception Test (TAT)** - A projective psychological test involving the interpretation of ambiguous pictures, used to assess a person's social and emotional functioning.
11. **Transcranial Magnetic Stimulation (TMS)** - A non-invasive procedure using magnetic fields to stimulate nerve cells in the brain, primarily used to treat depression.
12. **Token Economy** - A form of behaviour modification using incentives like tokens or points to reinforce positive behaviour, often used in therapeutic settings.

These definitions provide a general overview, and symptoms or experiences can differ from person to person.

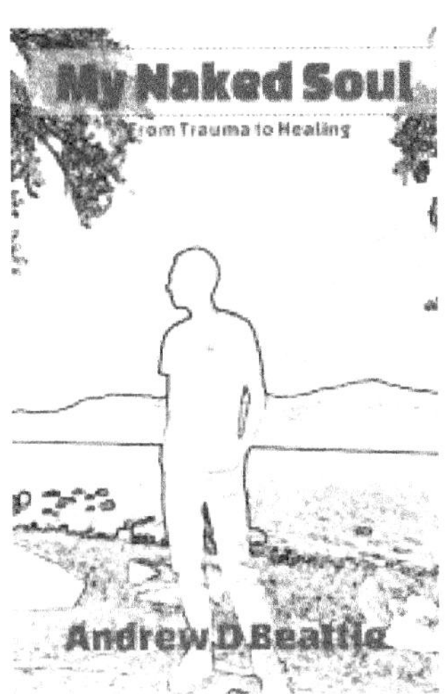
My Naked Soul
From Trauma to Healing
Andrew D Beattie

Chapter 21: U is for...

———

1. **Unipolar Depression** - A term sometimes used to describe Major Depressive Disorder to differentiate it from Bipolar Disorder, which includes both depressive and manic episodes.
2. **Unconscious** - The part of the mind that contains thoughts, memories, and desires that are not currently in conscious awareness but can influence behaviour.
3. **Utilitarianism** - A philosophical theory often discussed in ethics of healthcare, which suggests the best action is the one that maximizes utility or happiness.
4. **Undoing** - A psychological defence mechanism where a person tries to 'undo' an unhealthy, destructive, or otherwise threatening thought or action by engaging in contrary behaviour.
5. **Uppers** - Slang term for stimulant drugs, which can include prescription medications like Adderall or illegal substances like cocaine; often misused for their mood-enhancing effects.
6. **Unconditioned Stimulus** - In classical conditioning, a stimulus that naturally triggers a response without needing to be learned.
7. **Ultradian Rhythm** - Biological rhythms that occur more than once each day, such as cycles of sleep architecture, which can be affected in some mental

health conditions.

8. **Universal Screening** - The practice of evaluating all individuals in a particular setting for a certain condition or disorder, often used in schools for behavioural and emotional screening.

9. **Unstructured Interview** - A type of interview where questions are not prearranged, often used in qualitative research in psychology.

10. **Unresolved Grief** - A complicated form of grief that is prolonged and affects normal functioning, often requiring therapeutic intervention.

11. **Uptake Inhibitor** - A type of drug that inhibits the reuptake of neurotransmitters like serotonin or dopamine, commonly used in treating conditions like depression and anxiety.

These definitions provide a general overview, and symptoms or experiences can differ from person to person.

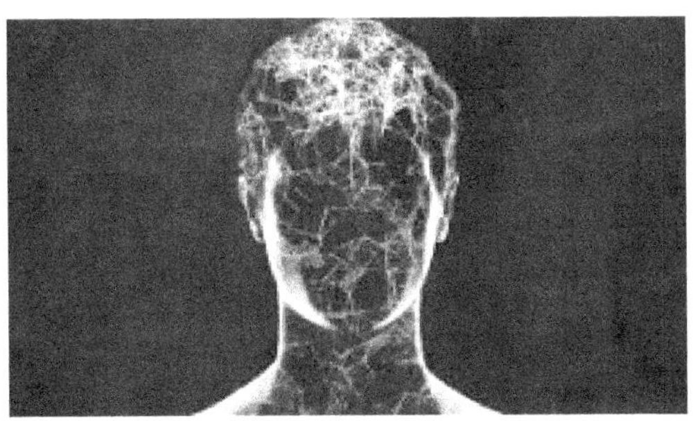

Chapter 22: V is for ...

———

1. **Validation** - The recognition and acceptance of another person's thoughts, feelings, or behaviours, often used as a therapeutic technique.
2. **Vicarious Trauma** - Emotional stress experienced when empathizing with a trauma victim's experience, often affecting caregivers and medical professionals.
3. **Venlafaxine** - An antidepressant medication in the serotonin-norepinephrine reuptake inhibitor (SNRI) class, commonly used to treat depression and anxiety disorders.
4. **Vagus Nerve** - A nerve that plays a role in regulating mood, heart rate, and other functions; sometimes stimulated as a treatment for depression.
5. **Vulnerability** - The quality or state of being exposed to emotional or physical risk, often discussed in the context of predispositions to mental health issues.
6. **Visual Hallucinations** - Seeing things that are not present, a symptom that can occur in various mental disorders like schizophrenia or during substance abuse.
7. **Vicodin** - A prescription pain medication containing hydrocodone and acetaminophen, sometimes abused for its calming effects, leading to potential mental health issues like dependency.
8. **Virtual Reality Exposure Therapy (VRET)** - A treatment that uses virtual reality technology to

expose patients to feared objects or scenarios as part of a therapeutic process, often for treating phobias or PTSD.

9. **Verbal Abuse** - The use of words to harm another individual, which can have long-term effects on emotional well-being.

10. **Volition** - The cognitive process by which an individual decides on and commits to a course of action, often discussed in mental health as it relates to impaired decision-making capabilities in some disorders.

11. **Vasopressin** - A hormone related to social behaviour, stress, and bonding; sometimes studied in relation to mental health issues like anxiety and depression.

These definitions provide a general overview, and symptoms or experiences can differ from person to person.

Chapter 23: W is for...

1. **Withdrawal** - The symptoms that occur after stopping the use of a substance to which one has become addicted.
2. **Well-being** - A state of overall health, happiness, and comfort, often a focus in mental health treatment and research.
3. **Worry** - The act of feeling anxious or concerned, often excessive in nature and a primary feature of anxiety disorders.
4. **Word Salad** - A symptom where speech is incoherent and disorganized, commonly seen in conditions like schizophrenia.
5. **White Matter** - The part of the brain that contains myelinated nerve fibres and is important for communication between different brain regions; often studied in relation to mental health conditions.
6. **Workaholism** - The condition of being addicted to work, often to the detriment of other aspects of one's life, including mental health.
7. **Willpower** - The ability to control one's actions, impulses, or emotions, often discussed in the context of addictive behaviours or impulse control disorders.
8. **Wish Fulfilment** - A psychological concept where dreams or actions are interpreted as the realization of unconscious desires, often explored in psychoanalytic theory.

9. **War Neurosis** - An older term for what is now often referred to as post-traumatic stress disorder (PTSD), specifically related to combat experience.
10. **Wernicke's Area** - A region of the brain involved in language comprehension, often studied in relation to speech disorders or conditions affecting communication.
11. **Working Memory** - A cognitive system responsible for temporarily holding and manipulating information, often impaired in disorders like ADHD.

These definitions provide a general overview, and symptoms or experiences can differ from person to person.

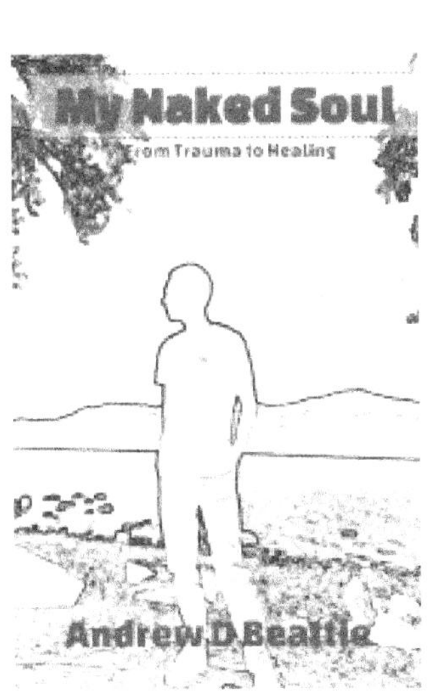

Chapter 24: X is for...

1. **Xanax** - A brand name for alprazolam, a medication used to treat anxiety and panic disorders.
2. **Xenophobia** - An intense or irrational fear or hatred of people from other countries or cultures, which can sometimes be a symptom or feature of certain mental health conditions.
3. **Xerostomia** - Dry mouth, which can be a side effect of various psychiatric medications, including antipsychotics and antidepressants.
4. **XYY Syndrome** - A chromosomal condition that may be associated with increased risk for learning disabilities and behavioural problems, although the link is not definitively established.
5. **X-Linked** - Referring to genes located on the X chromosome, sometimes discussed in the context of mental health when looking at genetic predispositions to certain conditions.

These definitions are general overviews, and symptoms or experiences can differ from person to person.

Chapter 25: Y is for...

1. **Yawning** - While a common behaviour, excessive yawning can sometimes be related to certain medical or psychiatric conditions, including anxiety or sleep disorders.

2. **Yerkes-Dodson Law** - A psychological principle stating that performance improves with increased arousal, but only up to a point, after which performance deteriorates.

3. **Yoga** - Although not strictly a medical term, yoga is increasingly studied and employed as a complementary treatment for various mental health conditions, such as depression and anxiety.

4. **Young Mania Rating Scale (YMRS)** - A commonly used diagnostic questionnaire that helps clinicians rate the severity of manic symptoms.

5. **Youth Risk Behaviour Surveillance System (YRBSS)** - A survey conducted to assess the prevalence of health-risk behaviours among young people, including mental health indicators like suicidal ideation.

6. **Yohimbine** - An alkaloid that is sometimes used to treat certain types of anxiety disorders but is more commonly known for its use in treating erectile dysfunction.

These definitions provide a general overview, and symptoms or experiences can differ from person to person.

Chapter 26: Z is for...

1. **Zoloft** - A brand name for sertraline, an antidepressant in the selective serotonin reuptake inhibitor (SSRI) class, commonly used to treat depression and anxiety disorders.
2. **Zyprexa** - A brand name for olanzapine, an antipsychotic medication commonly used to treat conditions like schizophrenia and bipolar disorder.
3. **Zeitgeber** - An external cue, such as light or temperature, that helps regulate biological rhythms, often discussed in the context of sleep disorders.
4. **Zen Meditation** - A form of meditation focusing on the breath and sometimes employed as a complementary treatment for mental health conditions like anxiety and depression.
5. **Zoning Out** - Informal term often used to describe a state of reduced awareness or distractibility; can be a symptom in conditions like ADHD or certain dissociative disorders.
6. **Zuclopenthixol** - An antipsychotic medication used to treat schizophrenia and other types of psychosis.

These definitions provide a general overview, and symptoms or experiences can differ from person to person.

PART TWO: The Importance of Treating Mental Health Conditions.

———

Treating mental health conditions is critical for enhancing an individual's overall quality of life. Effective treatment enables people to fully participate in social, occupational, and educational settings. Without proper care, mental health conditions can adversely affect physical health, manifesting in issues such as sleep disturbances or a weakened immune system.

Untreated mental health issues can also put a strain on personal relationships, potentially leading to social isolation. This can extend to impairing job performance, contributing to unemployment, and even posing safety risks to oneself or others.

Beyond the individual, untreated mental health conditions have wider economic repercussions, including lost workplace productivity and increased healthcare costs. By normalizing mental healthcare, we can also work toward reducing the societal stigma and discrimination that many individuals with mental health conditions face.

Moreover, early treatment is preventive; it can halt the progression of mental health issues and mitigate the severity of symptoms. Young people, in particular, may see their educational trajectory affected by untreated conditions, limiting their future opportunities.

Finally, some mental health conditions can lead to legal issues or a shortened lifespan if not adequately addressed. Therefore, treatment isn't just beneficial for the individual; it's crucial for society at large.

Chapter 27: A-Z of Treatment Options

1. **Antipsychotic Medication**: Used to manage symptoms of psychosis, such as hallucinations or delusions, often prescribed for conditions like schizophrenia.
2. **Art Therapy**: A form of expressive therapy that uses the creative process of making art to improve mental well-being.
3. **Biofeedback**: Teaches individuals how to control physiological functions through monitoring and feedback, often used for anxiety and stress-related conditions.
4. **Cognitive Behavioural Therapy (CBT)**: A form of psychotherapy that aims to change negative patterns of thinking, behaviour, or feelings.
5. **Counselling**: General term for talking therapies that treat mental health conditions, such as depression or anxiety, through conversation.
6. **Dialectical Behaviour Therapy (DBT)**: A form of CBT that focuses on mindfulness, emotional regulation, and interpersonal effectiveness, often used for borderline personality disorder.
7. **Electroconvulsive Therapy (ECT)**: A medical procedure where small electric currents are passed through the brain to treat severe depression and

other conditions.

8. **Exposure Therapy**: A type of behavioural therapy used to treat anxiety disorders by exposing the person to the source of their anxiety in a controlled setting.

9. **Family Therapy**: Addresses family dynamics that contribute to mental health conditions and involves family members in the therapeutic process.

10. **Group Therapy**: A type of psychotherapy that involves one or more therapists working with a group of individuals at the same time.

11. **Holistic Therapies**: Approaches like acupuncture, yoga, or dietary supplements that aim to treat the whole person, often used in conjunction with traditional treatments.

12. **Interpersonal Therapy (IPT)**: Focuses on improving interpersonal relationships and social functioning to help treat depression.

13. **Light Therapy**: Used for seasonal affective disorder (SAD) and certain other conditions, it involves exposure to artificial light.

14. **Medication**: Includes antidepressants, anxiolytics, and mood stabilizers used to treat various mental health conditions.

15. **Mindfulness-Based Cognitive Therapy (MBCT)**: Combines mindfulness strategies with CBT for treating depression and preventing relapse.

16. **Narrative Therapy**: Focuses on the stories people tell about their lives and aims to rewrite these narratives in a more positive way.

17. **Occupational Therapy**: Helps individuals perform

everyday tasks and improves their living skills, often used for conditions like PTSD or severe anxiety.

18. **Pharmacotherapy**: The use of medication to treat mental health disorders, often in conjunction with other treatments.

19. **Play Therapy**: Often used with children to help express their experiences and feelings through a natural, self-guided, self-healing process.

20. **Psychodynamic Therapy**: Explores unconscious processes and helps individuals understand the roots of emotional distress.

21. **Psychoeducation**: Educates individuals and families about mental health conditions and treatments, often used as a supplementary treatment.

22. **Psychotherapy**: General term for treating mental health problems by talking with a mental health provider.

23. **Reality Therapy**: Focuses on current issues affecting a person's life, teaching problem-solving and better decision-making.

24. **Recreational Therapy**: Uses activities like music and art to treat various mental health conditions, including emotional and cognitive issues.

25. **Support Groups**: Peer-led groups that provide a space for people with similar conditions to share experiences and coping strategies.

26. **Transcranial Magnetic Stimulation (TMS)**: A non-invasive procedure using magnetic fields to stimulate nerve cells in the brain, often used for depression.

27. **Virtual Reality Exposure Therapy (VRET)**: Uses

virtual environments to expose individuals to situations that trigger anxiety or PTSD.

These treatment options provide a range of approaches to managing mental health conditions and are often used in combination for more effective results. Always consult a healthcare provider for a tailored treatment plan.

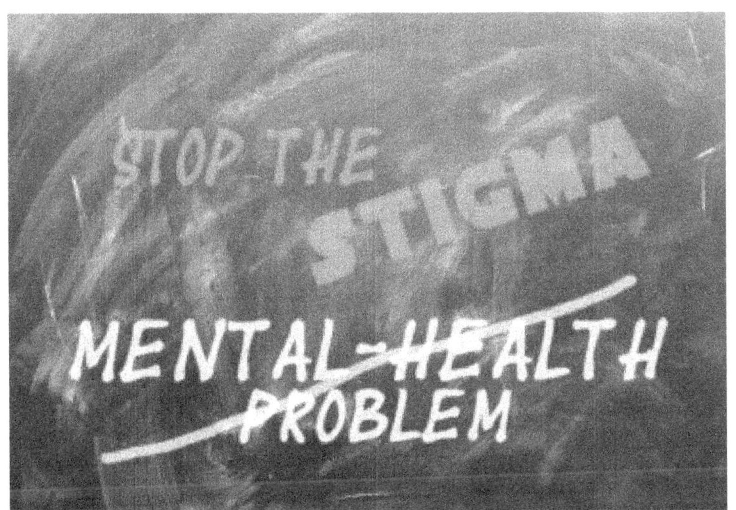

Chapter 28: Stigma

Societal attitudes toward mental health have certainly evolved over the years, with growing awareness and advocacy helping to bring mental health issues into mainstream conversations. Despite these strides, the stigma surrounding mental health persists, often rooted in misunderstandings, cultural norms, or a lack of education on the subject. This stigma manifests in various ways, including social discrimination, stereotyping, and marginalization of individuals with mental health conditions.

The lingering stigma often discourages people from seeking help due to fear of judgment or negative repercussions in their personal and professional lives. It can even affect policy and funding decisions, contributing to inadequate mental health services and support. Moreover, stigma can perpetuate harmful myths and assumptions about mental health conditions, leading to misdiagnosis, inappropriate treatment, and further isolation for those affected.

Combatting this stigma requires a multi-faceted approach:

Education

EDUCATIONAL PROGRAMS in schools and communities serve as one of the most effective ways to combat mental health stigma. By teaching young people about mental health from an early age, misconceptions can be corrected before they take root. Educational initiatives can also extend to adult learning platforms, community centers, and workplaces, reaching a broader audience.

Media Responsibility

MEDIA PLAYS A PIVOTAL role in shaping societal attitudes. Irresponsible portrayals that reinforce stereotypes can perpetuate stigma, while nuanced and accurate portrayals can enlighten the public. Journalists, writers, and filmmakers need to be educated on the subject and held accountable for how they depict mental health conditions.

Open Dialogue

BREAKING THE SILENCE around mental health issues is crucial. Employers can create spaces where employees feel safe discussing their mental health, while families can foster environments where it's okay to talk about emotional well-being. The more openly people discuss mental health, the less stigmatizing it becomes.

Peer Support

THE IMPORTANCE OF PEER support groups can't be overstated. These groups provide safe spaces for individuals to share experiences, seek advice, and offer emotional support. Peer-led organizations also have the advantage of "lived experience," making them relatable and trustworthy sources of help.

Legislation and Policy

GOVERNMENT AND ORGANIZATIONAL policies can either perpetuate or diminish stigma. Anti-discrimination laws can protect individuals with mental health conditions in various facets of life, including employment, housing, and healthcare. Companies can also adopt mental health-friendly policies, like flexible work hours or mental health days, to accommodate the needs of their employees.

Healthcare Training

DOCTORS, NURSES, THERAPISTS, and other healthcare providers are often the first point of contact for individuals seeking help for mental health issues. Proper training in diagnosing and treating mental health conditions is vital, as misdiagnosis or incorrect treatment can have dire consequences and reinforce stigma.

Celebrity Advocacy

CELEBRITIES AND PUBLIC figures who openly discuss their struggles with mental health help normalize the conversation on a large scale. Their stories can make a substantial impact, not just in raising awareness but also in reducing stigma, as they reach wide and diverse audiences.

Community Outreach

COMMUNITY EVENTS, WORKSHOPS, and mental health awareness campaigns can serve as effective grassroots methods for combating stigma. Direct interaction with community members can correct false information, validate the experiences of those with mental health conditions, and provide tangible resources for help.

By implementing these strategies across multiple sectors of society, we can create a more inclusive, understanding, and stigma-free environment for individuals dealing with mental health conditions. This, in turn, encourages more people to seek the treatment and support they need, benefiting society as a whole.

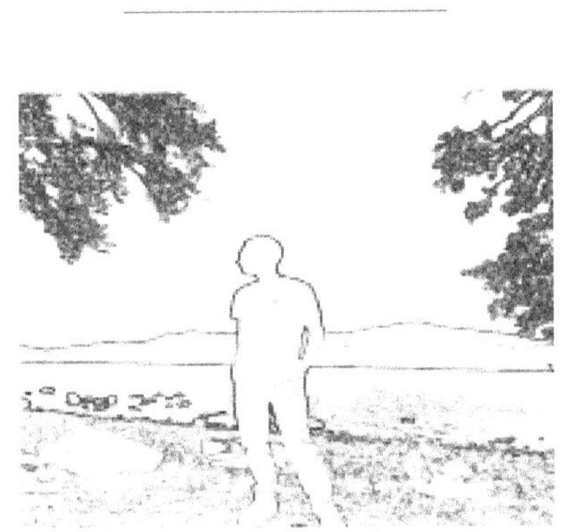

PART THREE : Mental Health Conditions

Cluster A personality disorders are a category of personality disorders characterized by odd, eccentric thinking or behavior. They include Paranoid Personality Disorder, Schizoid Personality Disorder, and Schizotypal Personality Disorder.

Cluster B personality disorders are characterized by dramatic, overly emotional, or unpredictable thinking and behavior. This cluster includes Borderline Personality Disorder, Narcissistic Personality Disorder, Histrionic Personality Disorder, and Antisocial Personality Disorder.

Cluster C personality disorders are characterized by anxious, fearful thinking or behavior. The disorders included in this cluster are Avoidant Personality Disorder, Dependent Personality Disorder, and Obsessive-Compulsive Personality Disorder (OCPD).

Chapter 29: Cluster A Conditions

Paranoid Personality Disorder

Paranoid Personality Disorder (PPD) is a mental health condition characterized by persistent and pervasive distrust and suspicion of others. People with PPD tend to view the actions of others as malevolent, even when there is no evidence to support these suspicions. This disorder falls under the "Cluster A" personality disorders, which are generally characterized by odd, eccentric thinking or behavior.

Core Features:

1. **Chronic Distrust**: A central feature of PPD is a deep-seated mistrust of others. This distrust often leads to social detachment and a reduced capacity for close relationships.
2. **Preoccupation with Hidden Motives**: Individuals with PPD tend to interpret other people's actions as deliberately deceitful, manipulative, or harmful, even when there's no rational basis for these beliefs.
3. **Hypervigilance**: Due to their constant suspicions, individuals with PPD are often on high alert for signs of betrayal or hostility, which can result in anxious or aggressive responses.
4. **Reluctance to Confide**: People with PPD often avoid sharing personal information with others due

to the fear that it will be used against them.

5. **Interpersonal Issues**: Relationships, both personal and professional, are often strained. Trust issues can make intimate relationships particularly difficult.

6. **Persistent Grudges**: Individuals with PPD may hold onto grudges for a long time, unwilling to forgive perceived slights or betrayals.

Diagnosis:

THE DIAGNOSIS TYPICALLY involves a comprehensive evaluation that may include interviews, questionnaires, and observation. Medical professionals usually rule out other potential causes for the symptoms, such as other personality disorders, mental health conditions, or medical issues.

Treatment:

TREATMENT CAN BE CHALLENGING, primarily because individuals with PPD have a hard time establishing trust with healthcare providers. However, psychotherapy or "talk therapy" can sometimes be effective. Medications are not generally used to treat the disorder itself but may be used to treat associated issues, like anxiety or depression.

Because of the enduring pattern of behavior and emotion that defines this disorder, treatment is often long-term and focuses on increasing coping mechanisms, enhancing social interaction skills, and challenging distorted thought patterns.

Understanding Paranoid Personality Disorder involves recognizing the depth and persistence of the distrust and suspicion that pervade the individual's worldview. While it can be a challenging condition to manage, appropriate psychological treatment can help improve quality of life for those affected.

Schizoid Personality Disorder

SCHIZOID PERSONALITY Disorder (SPD) is a mental health condition that falls under the "Cluster A" category of personality disorders, which are generally characterized by odd or eccentric behaviors. Unlike Paranoid Personality Disorder, which involves an excessive distrust of others, the defining feature of Schizoid Personality Disorder is a pervasive pattern of detachment from social relationships and a restricted range of emotional expression.

Core Features:

1. **Emotional Detachment**: Individuals with SPD often appear indifferent to the opportunity of forming close relationships and may even prefer spending time alone rather than with others.
2. **Limited Emotional Range**: People with this disorder often seem emotionally "flat" and may not derive much pleasure from activities that most people find enjoyable, including sexual activities.
3. **Social Isolation**: A preference for solitary activities and occupations often leads to social isolation, though the individual typically does not appear to be bothered by this isolation.
4. **Indifference to Praise or Criticism**: Unlike many

other personality disorders, individuals with SPD often appear indifferent to the opinions of others. They neither desire nor enjoy close relationships, including being a part of a family.

5. **Lack of Close Friends**: Apart from immediate family members, many people with SPD have no desire to form close friendships or romantic relationships, often seeming aloof, detached, and uninterested in other people.

Diagnosis:

THE DIAGNOSIS OF SCHIZOID Personality Disorder is typically made by a qualified mental health professional after a comprehensive psychological evaluation. This will usually include interviews and may also feature standardized tests or questionnaires. It's essential to rule out other potential causes for these symptoms, such as other mental health conditions, substance abuse, or medical issues.

Treatment:

TREATMENT FOR SPD CAN be quite challenging, partly because people with this disorder often do not see the need for treatment. They might not even be distressed by their symptoms unless they encounter a situation that requires social interaction or emotional expression.

1. **Psychotherapy**: Also known as talk therapy, psychotherapy can help individuals with SPD understand the emotions and behaviors affecting

their life.

2. **Medication**: While there are no medications specifically approved to treat SPD, medications like antipsychotic drugs or antidepressants may sometimes be used to treat symptoms that co-occur with this disorder, such as depression or anxiety.

3. **Coping Strategies**: Treatment might focus on helping individuals develop better social skills, improve their communication with others, and manage any co-occurring conditions like depression or anxiety.

Given the complexity and pervasiveness of the symptoms, long-term treatment is often required. Therapeutic goals generally aim at helping individuals form at least some relationships and engage in some activities, thereby improving their quality of life.

.

Schizotypal Personality Disorder

SCHIZOTYPAL PERSONALITY Disorder (STPD) is another condition within the Cluster A group of personality disorders, which are characterized by odd or eccentric behaviors. However, the central features of Schizotypal Personality Disorder are markedly different from those of Paranoid or Schizoid Personality Disorders. STPD is characterized by acute discomfort in social relationships, cognitive and perceptual distortions, and eccentric behavior.

Core Features:

1. **Peculiar Thinking**: Individuals with STPD often have unusual beliefs or "magical thinking," such as believing they can read other people's thoughts or that events contain special personal messages.
2. **Odd Behavior and Appearance**: Their appearance, speech, or behavior may be peculiar, leading them to be perceived as "weird" or "strange" by others. They might dress in unusual ways or have a very constricted or inappropriate emotional affect.
3. **Social Anxiety**: Despite a desire for intimacy and social connection, people with STPD often feel extremely anxious in social settings. This anxiety does not diminish as they become more familiar with people, making social interactions very challenging.
4. **Odd Speech**: Speech may be vague, overly elaborate, or inappropriately abstract, making communication difficult.
5. **Emotional Distance**: Like those with Schizoid Personality Disorder, individuals with STPD often appear distant and detached. However, this often stems from acute social anxiety rather than a lack of desire for social interaction.
6. **Suspiciousness or Paranoia**: Although not as intense as the distrust found in Paranoid Personality Disorder, people with STPD may still be overly suspicious of others.

Diagnosis:

DIAGNOSIS IS TYPICALLY made by a qualified mental health professional through a thorough evaluation that may include interviews, self-report questionnaires, and possibly additional diagnostic tests. It's important to rule out other mental disorders, as well as medical conditions or substance use that could contribute to these symptoms.

Treatment:

1. **Psychotherapy**: Cognitive-behavioral therapy (CBT) is often used to treat STPD. It helps the individual become aware of their thoughts, perceptions, and beliefs and challenges their validity.
2. **Medications**: Antipsychotic medications, as well as antidepressants and antianxiety medications, may be used to treat specific symptoms or co-occurring disorders.
3. **Social Skills Training**: Some individuals with STPD can benefit from social skills training, which teaches the nuances of social interaction and communication.
4. **Community Support**: Supportive community services, including case management and occupational therapy, can be beneficial.

SCHIZOTYPAL PERSONALITY Disorder can be a challenging condition to manage, but with effective treatment, many individuals can go on to lead fulfilling lives, albeit often with ongoing symptoms and limitations. The focus of treatment is typically on improving social functioning and reducing distorted thinking, thereby enhancing the individual's overall quality of life.

.

Commonalities in Treatment

FOR ALL CLUSTER A PERSONALITY disorders, a strong therapeutic relationship between the patient and healthcare provider is crucial. Consistent, long-term treatment is often necessary, and a multidisciplinary approach involving psychologists, psychiatrists, and social workers is typically the most effective.

It's important to note that while Cluster A disorders share some characteristics with psychotic disorders like schizophrenia, they are not as debilitating and are considered separate conditions. However, they may increase the risk of developing psychotic disorders later in life.

Chapter 30: Cluster B Conditions

Borderline Personality Disorder (BPD)

Borderline Personality Disorder (BPD) is a complex mental health disorder that falls under the "Cluster B" category of personality disorders, which are characterized by dramatic, emotional, or erratic behavior. BPD is distinct from other personality disorders in its intense emotional experiences, unstable relationships, and issues with self-image.

Core Features:

1. **Emotional Instability**: The rapid mood swings often make it difficult for individuals to maintain stable relationships or hold down a job. The emotional volatility can also lead to frequent changes in goals, career plans, and even sexual orientation.
2. **Fear of Abandonment**: This intense fear can result in desperate efforts to avoid being alone, which can include clinging to people who make them feel secure, as well as rejecting them pre-emptively to avoid being rejected first.
3. **Unstable Relationships**: The pattern of idealizing and then devaluing others can cycle rapidly and occur in all types of relationships, including friendships, family, and romantic relationships.
4. **Distorted Self-Image**: These distortions can also

manifest as chronic feelings of emptiness or boredom. People with BPD may lack a clear sense of who they are and can experience their identity as shifting or unstable.

5. **Impulsive Behaviors**: The impulsivity can extend to areas beyond substance abuse and can include impulsivity in decision-making, such as abruptly quitting a job or ending a relationship.

6. **Self-Harm and Suicidal Behavior**: These actions often serve as a way to manage intense emotional pain, and they can occur with little warning, often in response to real or perceived abandonment or rejection.

Additional Treatment Approaches:

1. **Transference-Focused Psychotherapy (TFP)**: This type of therapy focuses on the relationship between the patient and therapist to identify the distorted self-perception and interpersonal relations that individuals with BPD often experience.

2. **Schema Therapy**: This approach combines elements of CBT with other forms of psychotherapy and focuses on changing negative life patterns and self-beliefs that are resistant to treatment.

3. **Pharmacotherapy**: Antipsychotic medications can be used to treat symptoms like irritability and paranoid thoughts. Mood stabilizers can help regulate mood swings, and SSRIs (selective serotonin reuptake inhibitors) may help alleviate depression

and impulsivity.

4. **Integrated Treatment**: In some cases, a combination of therapies and medications is the most effective course of treatment, supplemented by case management to handle other life areas impacted by the disorder.

5. **Hospitalization**: In some severe cases involving self-harm or suicidal tendencies, inpatient care may be necessary.

Long-Term Outcomes:

IT'S WORTH NOTING THAT while BPD is often viewed as a challenging disorder to treat, there is considerable hope for those who seek comprehensive treatment. Over time, many people experience a significant reduction in symptoms and an improved quality of life. However, ongoing treatment and support are often necessary for maintaining these gains.

In essence, understanding and treating BPD is not a straightforward process. It often requires a multi-disciplinary approach and the involvement of family and loved ones for optimal outcomes.

Narcissistic Personality Disorder (NPD)

Narcissistic Personality Disorder (NPD) is a mental health condition characterized by a long-term pattern of exaggerated self-importance, an excessive need for admiration, and a lack of empathy toward others. It falls under the category of "Cluster B" personality disorders, which are generally marked by emotional, dramatic, or erratic behavior.

Narcissistic Personality Disorder (NPD) is a mental health condition characterized by a pervasive pattern of grandiosity, a deep need for excessive attention and admiration, and a lack of empathy for others. This condition is one of several personality disorders categorized in the Diagnostic and Statistical Manual of Mental Disorders (DSM-5), a classification tool used by mental health professionals. Here's a detailed look into its aspects:

The Clinical Picture

PEOPLE WITH NPD OFTEN display an inflated sense of their own importance and have a preoccupation with fantasies of unlimited success, power, and beauty. They believe that they're special and should only associate with equally special people. However, beneath this facade of ultra-confidence lies a fragile self-esteem, vulnerable to the slightest criticism.

Core Features:

Grandiosity:

PEOPLE WITH NPD HAVE an exaggerated sense of their own significance. They often believe that they have unique talents and should therefore be given special treatment. This sense of grandiosity can manifest in both their behavior and fantasies.

Need for Excessive Admiration:

THE SELF-ESTEEM OF individuals with NPD is often dependent on the admiration and validation they receive from others. They require constant praise and often expect others to comply with their wishes and ideas without questioning.

Lack of Empathy:

ONE OF THE MOST DISTINGUISHING features of NPD is a significant lack of empathy towards others. Individuals with NPD often find it difficult to recognize or understand others' needs and feelings, which can make interpersonal relationships challenging.

Sense of Entitlement:

THEY OFTEN EXPECT SPECIAL treatment and unquestioning compliance with their expectations. When these expectations are not met, it can result in rage or emotional withdrawal.

Exploitative Behavior:

IN THEIR QUEST FOR admiration and importance, people with NPD often exploit others without guilt or remorse. They will take advantage of other people's kindness or resources to achieve their own goals.

Envy and Belief That Others Are Envious:

PEOPLE WITH NPD OFTEN become envious of others' successes or possessions and believe that others are equally envious of them. This can result in feelings of entitlement to what others have, without recognizing their own shortcomings or the effort others have put into achieving something.

Fragile Self-esteem:

DESPITE THEIR OUTWARD appearance of confidence, people with NPD often have a very fragile sense of self-esteem and are highly sensitive to criticism. Any perceived attack on their grandiosity can result in significant emotional turmoil.

Treatment:

NPD IS CONSIDERED CHALLENGING to treat, primarily because people with this disorder often don't recognize that they have a problem. Treatment typically involves psychotherapy (commonly known as counseling or talk therapy), and medication may also be prescribed to treat associated symptoms like depression or anxiety.

Prognosis:

THE PROGNOSIS VARIES widely depending on the individual's willingness to seek and adhere to treatment. The condition can be lifelong but may become less severe as the individual ages.

Understanding NPD in depth is crucial for both the person suffering from the disorder and those around them, as its complex nature makes it difficult to manage and can have a significant impact on relationships and overall quality of life.

Histrionic Personality Disorder (HPD)

B personality disorders, according to the Diagnostic and Statistical Manual of Mental Disorders (DSM-5). It is marked by excessive emotionality, attention-seeking behavior, and a need for approval. Individuals with HPD are often dramatic, lively, and flirtatious and have a strong desire to be the center of attention in any social setting. Below are the core features and details of this disorder.

Core Features:

Excessive Emotionality:

PEOPLE WITH HPD OFTEN display an exaggerated level of emotions, sometimes akin to theatricality. This may include frequent expression of shallow, shifting emotions and overdramatic responses to events or situations.

Attention-Seeking Behavior:

A CONSTANT NEED FOR approval and attention characterizes those with HPD. They may use physical appearance, drama, or sexually provocative behavior to ensure they are the focus of others' attention.

Suggestibility:

INDIVIDUALS WITH HPD can be easily influenced by others or by current trends, displaying a lack of strong convictions or personal identity.

Shallow Expression of Emotions:

WHILE THEY ARE OFTEN highly emotive, the feelings may be surface-level and shifting, making it difficult for them to form deep, meaningful relationships.

Self-Centeredness:

THE INDIVIDUAL MAY be overly concerned with their own interests and have difficulty recognizing the needs and feelings of others.

Overly Concerned with Physical Appearance:

PEOPLE WITH HPD OFTEN invest excessive time and energy into their physical appearance to draw attention to themselves.

Dramatic, Impressionistic Speech:

THEIR WAY OF COMMUNICATING can be excessively emotional and lacking in detail. They may exaggerate events or situations for emotional impact.

Perceived Relationships as More Intimate Than They Are:

INDIVIDUALS WITH HPD may believe that their relationships are more intimate and meaningful than they actually are, mistaking casual relationships for deep emotional bonds.

Treatment:

THERAPEUTIC TREATMENT is typically the recommended course of action for HPD. Cognitive-behavioral therapy (CBT) is often effective in helping the individual become more aware of their thoughts, feelings, and behaviors and learning to analyze and adapt them. Medication may also be prescribed to manage specific symptoms, although it does not treat the disorder itself.

Prognosis:

THE PROGNOSIS FOR HPD can vary depending on a range of factors, including the individual's willingness to engage in treatment and the severity of their symptoms. While the condition itself can be enduring, therapeutic interventions can often help manage symptoms and improve social functioning.

Understanding Histrionic Personality Disorder is crucial for both those who have the disorder and the people around them. Its impacts can be wide-ranging, affecting personal relationships, work life, and overall emotional well-being.

Antisocial Personality Disorder (ASPD)

ANTISOCIAL PERSONALITY Disorder (ASPD) is a mental health condition classified within Cluster B of the Diagnostic and Statistical Manual of Mental Disorders (DSM-5). ASPD is persistent pattern of disregard for the rights of others, along with a lack of empathy and a willingness to manipulate or exploit people for personal gain. Below are the core features of this disorder:.

Core Features:

Disregard for Social Norms:

INDIVIDUALS WITH ASPD often engage in behaviors that are grounds for arrest, such as theft, vandalism, or physical assault. They display a general lack of adherence to social, ethical, or legal standards.

Deceitfulness:

DECEPTION FOR PERSONAL gain or pleasure is common. This may manifest as lying, using aliases, or conning others.

Impulsivity:

PEOPLE WITH ASPD FREQUENTLY act on a whim, without planning or considering the consequences for themselves or others.

Irritability and Aggressiveness:

THERE MAY BE FREQUENT instances of physical fights or assaults. Individuals often have a low tolerance for frustration and may lash out in anger.

Reckless Disregard for Safety:

BOTH THEIR SAFETY AND the safety of others are often neglected, manifesting in activities like reckless driving, substance abuse, or hazardous behavior.

Irresponsibility:

CONSISTENT IRRESPONSIBILITY in work and financial matters, such as failing to sustain a job or honor financial commitments, is typical.

Lack of Remorse:

AFTER HARMING, MISTREATING, or stealing from another person, individuals with ASPD often feel neither remorse nor guilt. They may rationalize the behavior, trivialize it, or express indifference.

Treatment:

TREATING ANTISOCIAL Personality Disorder is challenging, largely because individuals with ASPD often don't seek treatment on their own. Even when they do enter treatment, their manipulative tendencies can make therapeutic progress difficult. Various therapeutic approaches, such as Cognitive Behavioral Therapy (CBT) and dialectical behavior therapy (DBT), have been tried, often with limited success. Medication is generally not considered effective in treating the core aspects of the disorder, although it may be used to manage associated symptoms like aggression or impulsivity.

Prognosis:

THE PROGNOSIS FOR ASPD varies. While many individuals with ASPD find it difficult to maintain stable relationships and jobs, some manage to integrate into society, sometimes through careers that allow for their risk-taking and manipulative tendencies. However, ASPD is often associated with substance abuse, legal issues, and a higher risk of violent behavior, which can have severe consequences for the individual and society.

Understanding Antisocial Personality Disorder is essential not only for the individuals who have it but also for society at large, given its association with criminal activity and other forms of social disruption. Treatment, although challenging, can help manage some of the symptoms and reduce the negative impact on the individual and those around them.

Common Challenges in Treatment

- **Non-compliance**: Many individuals with Cluster B disorders may not believe they need treatment or may resist mental health interventions.
- **Co-occurring Disorders**: These conditions often co-occur with mood disorders, eating disorders, or substance abuse, which can complicate treatment.
- **Impact on Families**: The erratic or volatile behavior associated with Cluster B disorders can be challenging for families and partners, making relationship or family therapy a necessary component of a comprehensive treatment plan.

BY UNDERSTANDING THE complexities and interwoven challenges of Cluster B disorders, healthcare providers can tailor treatment plans that address both the symptoms and the underlying behavioral patterns. Effective treatment usually requires long-term intervention and a multi-pronged approach involving medication, psychotherapy, and lifestyle adjustments.

Chapter 31: Cluster C Conditions

Avoidant Personality Disorder

Characteristics

- **Hypersensitivity to Criticism**: Even mild criticism can have a devastating impact, leading to avoidance of social situations where criticism is possible.
- **Desire for Social Relationships**: Despite their avoidance, many do desire companionship and friendship but find the risks too emotionally painful.
- **"Safety Behaviors"**: Some individuals develop "safety behaviors" like only going out in public at certain times to avoid interactions.

Treatment

CBT is a standard treatment, but exposure therapy, where the individual is gradually introduced to feared situations, is also effective. Social skills training can further enhance treatment by helping build confidence in social settings.

Dependent Personality Disorder

Characteristics

- **Urgent Relationship Transitions**: If a close relationship ends, they may urgently seek another one to provide the care and support they seek.

- **High Tolerance for Poor Treatment**: Often, individuals will tolerate mistreatment or abuse to avoid being alone.
- **Difficulty with Everyday Decisions**: They may require an excessive amount of advice and reassurance to make everyday decisions.

Treatment

TREATMENT PLANS OFTEN involve helping the person become more autonomous and capable of making decisions independently. Assertiveness training can be part of therapy to enable the individual to express themselves more effectively.

Obsessive-Compulsive Personality Disorder (OCPD)

Characteristics

- **Hoarding Behaviors**: Though not always present, some individuals may engage in hoarding behaviors, convinced that they'll need the items in the future.
- **Overconscientiousness in Social Situations**: There's often an overemphasis on "rules," which can make social interactions tense and formal.
- **Overwork**: A preoccupation with productivity often leads to overwork and neglect of leisure activities and friendships.

Treatment

CBT OFTEN FOCUSES ON cognitive restructuring, enabling the individual to identify and change the dysfunctional beliefs underlying their actions. Mindfulness and relaxation techniques may also be used to help manage perfectionistic tendencies.

Common Challenges in Treatment

- **Dual Diagnosis**: As Cluster C disorders often co-occur with anxiety and mood disorders, treating the co-occurring condition is crucial.
- **Therapeutic Alliance**: A strong therapeutic alliance is essential but may take time to establish, particularly for those with Avoidant Personality Disorder who may be inherently distrustful.
- **Long-term Treatment**: Due to the ingrained nature of the thought patterns, long-term treatment is often necessary.

A COMPREHENSIVE TREATMENT approach, involving a mix of psychotherapy, medication for co-occurring conditions, and lifestyle interventions, is generally the most effective strategy. By better understanding the complexities of Cluster C personality disorders, mental health providers can better tailor their interventions to meet the unique challenges each disorder presents.

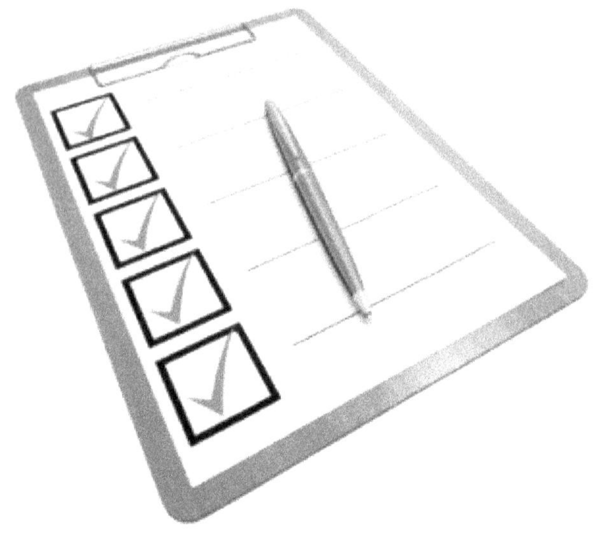

Chapter 32: Non-Cluster Conditions

Mental health conditions span a wide range, and not all of them fit neatly into the Cluster A, B, or C personality disorder categories as defined by the DSM-5 (Diagnostic and Statistical Manual of Mental Disorders). Here are some other categories and examples:

Mood Disorders

THESE DISORDERS PRIMARILY involve disturbances in a person's mood. Over the past few decades, there has been a considerable amount of research in treating mood disorders with medications like SSRIs, as well as psychotherapy such as Cognitive Behavioral Therapy (CBT).

- **Major Depressive Disorder**: Often involves a range of physical symptoms like changes in appetite and sleep and may also include suicidal thoughts.
- **Bipolar Disorder**: This disorder is particularly challenging because it involves mood swings that can affect judgment, concentration, and interpersonal relationships. Treatment often includes mood stabilizers like lithium.

Anxiety Disorders

ANXIETY DISORDERS ARE among the most common mental health conditions and are often comorbid with other mental health conditions like depression or OCD.

- **Generalized Anxiety Disorder (GAD)**: Medication and psychotherapy, particularly CBT, are common treatment routes.
- **Panic Disorder**: These attacks can be so severe that individuals may feel like they are dying, leading to avoidance behaviors.

Obsessive-Compulsive and Related Disorders

OBSESSIVE-COMPULSIVE and Related Disorders is a category of mental health conditions defined in the Diagnostic and Statistical Manual of Mental Disorders (DSM-5). These disorders are characterized by the presence of obsessions, compulsions, or both, which are time-consuming and distressing for the individual. Here are some of the core features and details about these disorders:

Core Disorders in this Category:

Obsessive-Compulsive Disorder (OCD):

OCD FEATURES RECURRING, unwanted thoughts (obsessions) and/or repetitive behaviors or mental acts (compulsions). For example, a person may fear contamination and engage in repetitive handwashing.

Body Dysmorphic Disorder:

THIS DISORDER INVOLVES obsessive thinking about one or more perceived flaws in physical appearance, which may not be noticeable to others.

Hoarding Disorder:

INDIVIDUALS WITH THIS disorder have persistent difficulty parting with possessions, regardless of their actual value, leading to clutter that disrupts their ability to use their living space.

Trichotillomania (Hair-Pulling Disorder):

THIS INVOLVES RECURRENT pulling out of one's hair, leading to hair loss and functional impairment.

Excoriation (Skin-Picking) Disorder:

PEOPLE WITH THIS DISORDER repeatedly pick at their skin, resulting in skin lesions and significant distress or impairment.

Common Features:

- **Obsessions:** Intrusive, unwanted, and distressing thoughts, images, or urges.
- **Compulsions:** Repetitive behaviors or mental acts performed to reduce the anxiety or distress associated

with obsessions.

- **Time-Consuming:** The obsessions and/or compulsions consume a significant amount of time, often more than one hour per day.
- **Distress or Impairment:** The symptoms cause significant distress or impairment in social, occupational, or other important areas of functioning.

Treatment Options:

THE PRIMARY TREATMENT options include:

- **Cognitive Behavioral Therapy (CBT):** Specifically, Exposure and Response Prevention (ERP) has been found effective in treating OCD.
- **Medication**: SSRIs and certain other types of medications are commonly used.
- **Combination**: Often, a combination of therapy and medication is the most effective treatment approach.
-

Prognosis:

THE COURSE OF OBSESSIVE-compulsive and related disorders can vary significantly between individuals. Some people may achieve good control of their symptoms through treatment, while others may continue to experience significant impairment.

Understanding these disorders is crucial for both diagnosis and treatment. Effective treatments are available, and early intervention often leads to better outcomes.

Post-Traumatic Stress Disorder (PTSD)

POST-TRAUMATIC STRESS Disorder (PTSD) is a mental health condition that can develop after an individual has been exposed to a traumatic event. Unlike personality disorders, PTSD is not classified under any cluster in the Diagnostic and Statistical Manual of Mental Disorders (DSM-5). It falls under the category of Trauma- and Stressor-Related Disorders. Here are the core features and other relevant information about PTSD:

Core Features:

Exposure to Traumatic Event:

THE ONSET OF PTSD SYMPTOMS typically follows exposure to actual or threatened death, serious injury, or sexual violence. This can happen through direct experience, witnessing it happening to someone else, or learning that a close family or friend was exposed to trauma.

Intrusive Symptoms:

INDIVIDUALS WITH PTSD often experience unwanted, distressing memories of the traumatic event, nightmares, and flashbacks, where it feels like the event is happening again.

Avoidance:

PEOPLE SUFFERING FROM PTSD often go to great lengths to avoid reminders of the trauma, which could be places, people, conversations, or activities that bring back memories of the event.

Negative Changes in Thoughts and Mood:

A PERSISTENT NEGATIVE emotional state, diminished interest in activities, feelings of detachment from others, and an inability to experience positive emotions are common.

Heightened Arousal:

SYMPTOMS MIGHT ALSO include irritability, outbursts of anger, reckless or self-destructive behavior, hypervigilance, an exaggerated startle response, and difficulties in concentration or sleep.

Treatment:

TREATMENT FOR PTSD generally involves psychotherapy, medication, or a combination of both. Cognitive Behavioral Therapy (CBT), including specific subtypes like exposure therapy and cognitive restructuring, has been found to be effective. Medication such as selective serotonin reuptake inhibitors (SSRIs) and serotonin-norepinephrine reuptake inhibitors (SNRIs) are commonly used for treatment as well.

Prognosis:

WHILE SOME PEOPLE MAY recover from PTSD over time, others may experience symptoms for many years if not treated. Treatment can help manage symptoms, improve quality of life, and provide coping strategies.

Understanding PTSD is crucial for both those who suffer from it and for society at large. The condition can significantly impair an individual's daily life, but with the right treatment and support, it's possible to manage the symptoms and lead a fulfilling life.

Neurodevelopmental Disorders

NEURODEVELOPMENTAL disorders are a group of conditions that typically manifest early in development and feature developmental deficits that produce impairments of personal, social, academic, or occupational functioning. These disorders are generally diagnosed in childhood but often continue into adulthood. Below are some core types of neurodevelopmental disorders and their defining features:

Core Disorders in this Category:

Attention-Deficit/Hyperactivity Disorder (ADHD):

ADHD IS CHARACTERIZED by ongoing patterns of inattention, hyperactivity, and/or impulsivity that interfere with functioning or development.

Autism Spectrum Disorders (ASD):

ASD INCLUDES A RANGE of conditions characterized by challenges with social interaction, verbal and nonverbal communication, and repetitive behaviors.

Intellectual Disability:

PREVIOUSLY REFERRED to as mental retardation, this disorder is characterized by limitations in intellectual functioning and adaptive behavior.

Learning Disorders:

THESE INCLUDE CONDITIONS like dyslexia, dyscalculia, and dysgraphia, which are characterized by difficulties in learning basic academic skills such as reading, writing, or arithmetic.

Motor Disorders:

CONDITIONS LIKE DEVELOPMENTAL Coordination Disorder, Tic Disorders (including Tourette's Syndrome), and Stereotypic Movement Disorder fall under this category.

Communication Disorders:

THESE INCLUDE CONDITIONS like childhood-onset fluency disorder (stuttering), language disorder, and social communication disorder.

Common Features:

- **Early Onset**: Symptoms usually manifest in the developmental period, often before the child enters school.
- **Functional Impairment**: The symptoms often result in significant challenges in social, occupational, or other important areas of functioning.
- **Varied Severity**: Disorders may be mild, moderate, or severe, depending on the level of impairment.

Treatment Options:

- **Behavioral Therapies**: These are often the first line of treatment, especially for ADHD and autism.
- **Educational Interventions**: Individualized Education Plans (IEPs) can be crucial for academic success.
- **Medication**: Medicines like stimulants for ADHD or antipsychotics for severe issues related to autism can be used.
- **Family Support**: Training for families to manage the challenges associated with these disorders can be beneficial.

Prognosis:

THE PROGNOSIS IS HIGHLY variable and depends on the specific disorder, its severity, and the availability and effectiveness of interventions.

It's crucial to recognize that while neurodevelopmental disorders often present significant challenges, many individuals with these conditions are able to lead fulfilling, productive lives, particularly when they receive timely and appropriate support and intervention.

Psychotic Disorders

PSYCHOTIC DISORDERS are mental health conditions characterized by distorted thinking, perception, emotions, language, sense of self, and behavior. People with psychotic disorders often experience a disconnection from reality that can include hallucinations, delusions, or thought disorders. Here are the core disorders in this category, along with their defining features:

Core Disorders in this Category:

Schizophrenia:

THE MOST WELL-KNOWN psychotic disorder, schizophrenia is characterized by a combination of hallucinations, delusions, and disorganized thinking and speech. Negative symptoms like anhedonia (loss of pleasure) and cognitive symptoms like impaired memory may also be present.

Schizoaffective Disorder:

THIS CONDITION IS A mix of symptoms of schizophrenia and mood disorders (either bipolar or depressive disorders).

Patients experience both psychotic symptoms and severe mood swings.

Delusional Disorder:

UNLIKE SCHIZOPHRENIA, individuals with delusional disorder experience delusions but don't typically have hallucinations, disorganized speech, or severe disorganized or catatonic behavior.

Brief Psychotic Disorder:

THIS DISORDER INVOLVES sudden onset of psychotic symptoms that last for at least a day but less than a month, followed by a full return to baseline functioning.

Other Specified and Unspecified Psychotic Disorders:

THESE CATEGORIES ARE used for conditions that don't neatly fit into the other categories of psychotic disorders.

Common Features:

- **Hallucinations**: These are false perceptions, such as hearing voices or seeing things that aren't present.
- **Delusions**: These are false beliefs strongly held despite contrary evidence, often paranoid (belief that others are plotting against the individual), grandiose, or bizarre.
- **Disorganized Thinking**: This can manifest as

trouble concentrating, following a conversation or remembering things, and can also involve disorganized or abnormal motor behavior.

Treatment Options:

- **Antipsychotic Medication**: Medicines are often the first line of treatment to alleviate symptoms.
- **Psychotherapy**: Cognitive-behavioral therapy (CBT) can be effective in treating symptoms and improving quality of life.
- **Social Support**: Support from loved ones and community resources is crucial for recovery and management.
- **Hospitalization**: This may be necessary in severe cases to stabilize the patient.

Prognosis:

THE COURSE OF PSYCHOTIC disorders can vary widely. Schizophrenia is often chronic and can be debilitating, but many people with psychotic disorders are able to function well with appropriate treatment and support.

Early identification and intervention significantly improve the prognosis, but it's generally a long-term treatment requiring ongoing medical and psychological care.

Eating Disorders

EATING DISORDERS ARE complex mental health conditions that involve preoccupations with food, body weight, and shape, leading to dangerous and often life-threatening eating behaviors. These disorders can significantly impact physical health and can co-occur with other mental health conditions like anxiety disorders, substance abuse, or depression. Here are some of the core types of eating disorders along with their defining features:

Core Types:

Anorexia Nervosa:

PEOPLE WITH ANOREXIA nervosa see themselves as overweight, even if they're underweight. They weigh themselves frequently, eat very small quantities, and avoid certain foods or meals altogether. Severe restriction of food intake leads to malnourishment and a host of physical problems.

Bulimia Nervosa:

INDIVIDUALS WITH BULIMIA nervosa eat large amounts of food in short periods, followed by behaviors to avoid weight gain such as forced vomiting, excessive use of laxatives, or extreme exercising. Unlike anorexia, people with bulimia may maintain a "normal" weight, but the psychological and physical effects are equally damaging.

Binge-Eating Disorder:

PEOPLE WITH THIS DISORDER lose control over their eating, similar to bulimia, but do not regularly engage in purging, excessive exercise, or fasting. As a result, many individuals with binge-eating disorder are overweight or obese.

Pica:

IN THIS LESS COMMON eating disorder, individuals consume non-food substances like soap, cloth, and hair. This can lead to a range of health problems, including poisoning, intestinal problems, and nutritional deficiencies.

Other Specified Feeding or Eating Disorders (OSFED):

THIS IS A CATEGORY for disorders that don't neatly fit into the above categories but still represent significant and dangerous disturbances in eating behavior.

Common Features:

- **Preoccupation with Food, Dieting, and Body Size**: Individuals are often obsessed with food, dieting, and body image, spending an inordinate amount of time thinking about these subjects.
- **Emotional and Psychological Distress**: Eating disorders are often accompanied by feelings of guilt, shame, and anxiety, usually around eating or meal times.
- **Physical Health Risks**: These can include heart problems, digestive issues, bone loss, and in severe cases, death.

Treatment Options:

- **Psychological Therapy**: Cognitive-behavioral therapy (CBT) is often considered the most effective form of treatment for eating disorders.
- **Medical Treatment**: This can include hospitalization for severe malnutrition or complications.
- **Nutritional Counseling**: Dietary plans are often part of the treatment process.

- **Medications**: Antidepressants or antianxiety medications can sometimes be used alongside other treatments, but there is limited evidence for their efficacy in treating eating disorders alone.

EATING DISORDERS ARE often chronic and can be difficult to treat, requiring a multi-disciplinary approach that may involve doctors, psychologists, and dietitians. The sooner they are identified and treated, the better the chances for recovery.

Chapter 33: Adult-Onset Conditions

A dult-onset mental health issues refer to psychiatric disorders that first manifest in adulthood, typically after the age of 18. It's worth noting that some mental health conditions can and do appear for the first time in adulthood, even if the individual had no significant mental health concerns earlier in life. Conditions that can have adult onset include, but are not limited to:

Mood Disorders

MOOD DISORDERS ARE a category of mental health conditions characterized primarily by disturbances in a person's emotional state. These disturbances can manifest as periods of intense sadness, excessive joy, or fluctuations between the two. Mood disorders can significantly interfere with an individual's daily life, affecting their ability to work, maintain relationships, and even carry out basic tasks. Here's a more detailed look:

Core Types:

Major Depressive Disorder (MDD):

IN MDD, SYMPTOMS INCLUDE persistent sadness, lack of interest in activities, fatigue, and feelings of worthlessness or guilt. This disorder may lead to physical problems, such as sleep disturbances and changes in appetite, as well as severe impairments in daily functioning.

Bipolar Disorder:

ALSO KNOWN AS MANIC-depressive illness, this condition involves episodes of extreme mood swings, ranging from depressive lows to manic highs. Manic episodes might involve increased energy, reduced need for sleep, and risky behavior, while depressive episodes are characterized by low energy, sadness, and lack of interest in activities.

Dysthymia (Persistent Depressive Disorder):

THIS IS A CHRONIC FORM of depression, but the symptoms are less severe than in major depressive disorder. However, because of its long-lasting nature, people may find it just as disabling.

Cyclothymic Disorder:

THIS IS A MILDER FORM of bipolar disorder. People with cyclothymia experience chronic fluctuations in mood that are less severe than those in full-blown bipolar disorder.

Seasonal Affective Disorder (SAD):

DEPRESSIVE EPISODES that occur at a specific time of year, usually in winter, characterize this disorder. It's believed that the lack of sunlight contributes to the symptoms of SAD.

Common Features:

- **Emotional Symptoms**: Feelings of sadness, emptiness, or elevated mood are common.
- **Cognitive Impairments**: Concentration, decision-making, and memory may be affected.
- **Physical Symptoms**: Sleep disturbances, changes in appetite, and fatigue are often present.

Treatment Options:

- **Pharmacotherapy**: Antidepressants like SSRIs and mood stabilizers such as lithium are commonly prescribed.
- **Psychotherapy**: Cognitive Behavioral Therapy (CBT), Interpersonal Therapy (IPT), and other talk therapies are often effective.
- **Lifestyle Changes**: Exercise, proper nutrition, and stress management can support medical treatments.
- **Electroconvulsive Therapy (ECT)**: Used in severe, life-threatening cases or when other treatments have failed.

UNDERSTANDING THE NUANCES of mood disorders is critical for effective treatment, which usually involves a combination of medication and psychotherapy. Early intervention often leads to better outcomes.

Anxiety Disorders

ANXIETY DISORDERS ARE a group of mental health conditions characterized by excessive and persistent worry, fear, or anxiety that interferes with daily activities. These disorders go beyond temporary worry or fear; the anxiety does not go away and can worsen over time. Below is a detailed look at anxiety disorders:

Core Types:

Generalized Anxiety Disorder (GAD):

IN GAD, INDIVIDUALS experience excessive, long-lasting anxiety and worry about various aspects of life, including work, health, and relationships. The anxiety often lacks a specific focus or trigger.

Panic Disorder:

CHARACTERIZED BY FREQUENT, sudden attacks of intense fear and physical symptoms that can include chest pain, heart palpitations, and shortness of breath. These episodes are often triggered by stress or specific situations.

Social Anxiety Disorder (Social Phobia):

A FEAR OF SOCIAL SITUATIONS where the individual could be scrutinized or judged by others. The anxiety can interfere with daily routines and may lead to avoidance of social settings.

Specific Phobias:

INTENSE, IRRATIONAL fears triggered by specific objects or situations, such as spiders, heights, or flying. The level of fear is usually disproportionate to the actual threat or danger.

Obsessive-Compulsive Disorder (OCD):

ALTHOUGH SOMETIMES categorized separately, OCD features repetitive, distressing thoughts and ritualistic behaviors designed to reduce anxiety. These rituals, however, provide only temporary relief.

Post-Traumatic Stress Disorder (PTSD):

TRIGGERED BY EXPERIENCING or witnessing a terrifying event, PTSD is characterized by flashbacks, nightmares, and severe anxiety, along with uncontrollable thoughts about the event.

Common Features:

- **Emotional Symptoms**: Excessive worry, fear, feeling of impending doom.
- **Cognitive Impairments**: Rumination, anticipation of worst-case scenarios, and dread.
- **Physical Symptoms**: Sweating, trembling, dizziness,

rapid heart rate.

Treatment Options:

- **Pharmacotherapy**: Anti-anxiety medications like benzodiazepines, SSRIs, and other antidepressants are often prescribed.
- **Psychotherapy**: Cognitive Behavioral Therapy (CBT) is the most effective form of therapy for treating anxiety disorders.
- **Lifestyle Changes**: Mindfulness, meditation, and relaxation techniques can also help manage symptoms.
- **Exposure Therapy**: Particularly useful for specific phobias and social anxiety disorder.

IT'S CRUCIAL TO GET a proper diagnosis and treatment plan tailored to the individual's needs, as untreated anxiety disorders can lead to a diminished quality of life. Early intervention often provides the best chance for successful treatment.

Psychotic Disorders

PSYCHOTIC DISORDERS are a group of severe mental health conditions characterized by distorted awareness and thinking. These disorders typically involve hallucinations, delusions, or disorganized thinking that can significantly impair perception, judgment, and ability to function in daily life. Below are some details about psychotic disorders:

Core Types:

Schizophrenia:

THIS IS ONE OF THE most well-known psychotic disorders. It involves a range of cognitive, behavioral, and emotional dysfunctions, including hallucinations, delusions, and impaired insight.

Schizoaffective Disorder:

THIS DISORDER IS A hybrid of schizophrenia and a mood disorder like bipolar disorder or depression. Individuals experience symptoms of both psychosis and mood disturbance.

Delusional Disorder:

IN THIS DISORDER, INDIVIDUALS experience delusions but don't have the hallucinations, thought disorder, or mood symptoms seen in schizophrenia.

Brief Psychotic Disorder:

CHARACTERIZED BY SUDDEN and short bouts of psychotic behavior, often in response to a very stressful event, such as bereavement.

Substance/Medication-Induced Psychotic Disorder:

THIS IS A FORM OF PSYCHOSIS that is triggered by the use of or withdrawal from drugs or medications.

Common Features:

- **Hallucinations**: Sensory experiences that occur without any stimulus. Auditory hallucinations (hearing voices) are most common.
- **Delusions**: Strongly held false beliefs that are resistant to reasoning or confrontation with actual facts.
- **Disorganized Thinking**: Individuals may have trouble organizing their thoughts or connecting them logically. Speech may be hard to follow.
- **Negative Symptoms**: Emotional flatness, lack of pleasure in everyday life, lack of ability to initiate and sustain activities.
- **Cognitive Symptoms**: Problems with attention, certain types of memory, and executive functions like planning are common.

Treatment Options:

- **Pharmacotherapy**: Antipsychotic medications are the mainstay of treatment, aiming to control symptoms.
- **Psychotherapy**: Cognitive Behavioral Therapy (CBT) for psychosis, supportive therapy, and family

education can be helpful adjuncts to medication.

- **Hospitalization**: In severe cases, or if there's a risk of harm to oneself or others, hospitalization may be necessary.
- **Community Support**: Social skills training, vocational rehabilitation, and supported employment can help with social and occupational functioning.

UNDERSTANDING AND TREATING psychotic disorders is complex, and it often involves a multi-faceted approach that includes healthcare providers, mental health professionals, and support from family and community. Early diagnosis and treatment are crucial for better long-term outcomes.

Personality Disorders

PERSONALITY DISORDERS are a group of mental health conditions characterized by enduring patterns of behavior, cognition, and inner experience, which deviate markedly from the expectations of the individual's culture. These patterns are pervasive, inflexible, and often lead to distress or impairment in social, occupational, or other important areas of functioning. Here are some details:

Core Types:

Cluster A (Odd or Eccentric Disorders)

- **Paranoid Personality Disorder**: Marked by

persistent distrust and suspicion of others.

- **Schizoid Personality Disorder**: Characterized by detachment from social relationships and limited emotional expression.
- **Schizotypal Personality Disorder**: Involves eccentric behavior, distorted thinking, and discomfort with close relationships.

Cluster B (Dramatic, Emotional or Erratic Disorders)

- **Antisocial Personality Disorder**: Persistent pattern of violating the rights of others, lack of empathy.
- **Borderline Personality Disorder**: Features instability in emotions, self-image, and interpersonal relationships.
- **Histrionic Personality Disorder**: Excessive attention-seeking and emotionally dramatic behavior.
- **Narcissistic Personality Disorder**: Long-term pattern of exaggerated self-importance and a lack of empathy.

Cluster C (Anxious or Fearful Disorders)

- **Avoidant Personality Disorder**: Extreme social inhibition and sensitivity to negative evaluation.
- **Dependent Personality Disorder**: Excessive need to be cared for, leading to submissive and clinging behavior.
- **Obsessive-Compulsive Personality Disorder**:

Preoccupation with orderliness, perfectionism, and control.

Common Features:

- **Enduring Patterns**: These are long-standing ways of behaving and relating to others, often beginning in adolescence or early adulthood.
- **Impairment**: These patterns often lead to significant distress or disability in social, occupational, or other important functions.
- **Stability Over Time**: Symptoms are stable over time and across situations.
- **Ego-Syntonic Nature**: Many individuals with personality disorders don't recognize that their behaviors are problematic, which often leads to conflicts with others.

Treatment Options:

- **Psychotherapy**: Dialectical Behavior Therapy (DBT), Cognitive Behavioral Therapy (CBT), and other psychotherapeutic approaches are often effective.
- **Pharmacotherapy**: Medication like antidepressants or antipsychotics may be used to treat co-occurring conditions or specific symptoms.
- **Support Groups**: Peer-led groups can offer social support and understanding that may not be available elsewhere.

- **Family and Social Support**: Educating and involving families can be vital, as relationship difficulties are often central to the disorder.

PERSONALITY DISORDERS are complex and often require a tailored and multi-disciplinary approach for effective treatment. Early intervention and a commitment to long-term treatment can lead to better outcomes.

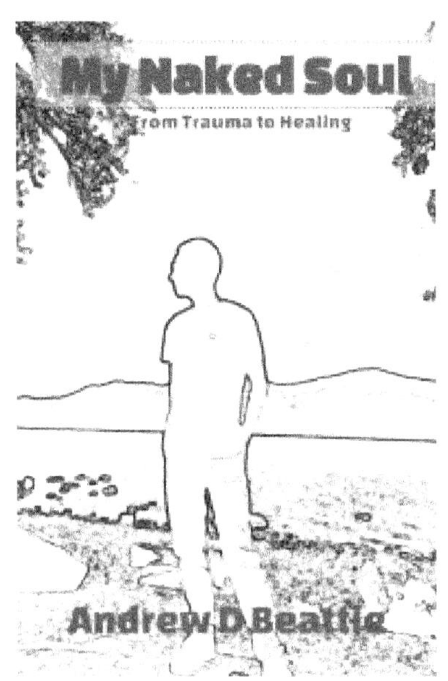

My Naked Soul
From Trauma to Healing
Andrew D Beattie

Other Disorders

Obsessive-Compulsive Disorder (OCD)

Core Features:

- **Obsessions**: Unwanted and distressing thoughts, images, or urges that repeatedly enter one's mind, triggering feelings of anxiety or discomfort.
- **Compulsions**: Ritualistic behaviors or mental acts that a person feels compelled to perform to alleviate the distress caused by obsessions.

Onset:

- **Childhood**: Early onset is often more severe and may be accompanied by other psychiatric conditions like ADHD or tics.
- **Adolescence**: Hormonal changes and life stressors like school can trigger the onset or exacerbation of symptoms.
- **Adulthood**: While less common, OCD can start in adulthood, often triggered by stress, major life changes, or health concerns.

Treatment Options:

- **Cognitive Behavioral Therapy (CBT):** Specifically, Exposure and Response Prevention (ERP) is the most effective form of CBT for OCD.
- **Pharmacotherapy:** SSRIs like fluoxetine and fluvoxamine are often used.
- **Support Groups:** Peer support can be very helpful in dealing with the day-to-day challenges of OCD.

Post-Traumatic Stress Disorder (PTSD)

Core Features:

- **Intrusion:** Intrusive thoughts, nightmares, and flashbacks of the traumatic event.
- **Avoidance:** Avoiding places, people, and activities that remind the person of the traumatic event.
- **Negative Alterations in Cognitions and Mood:** Feelings of detachment, negative emotional states, distorted blame of self or others.
- **Increased Arousal Symptoms:** Irritability, reckless behavior, hypervigilance, and

heightened startle response.

Onset:

- Can develop at any age following exposure to a traumatic event like violence, natural disasters, or severe accidents.
- **Acute Stress Disorder**: Symptoms occurring within 4 weeks of the traumatic event may precede PTSD.
- **Delayed Onset**: Sometimes, symptoms may not appear until years after the traumatic event.

Treatment Options:

- **Trauma-focused CBT**: Helps individuals confront and reframe their thoughts about the trauma.
- **Eye Movement Desensitization and Reprocessing (EMDR)**: Focuses on processing and making sense of the traumatic memories.
- **Pharmacotherapy**: Antidepressants like SSRIs and SNRIs are often used.
- **Support Groups**: Peer-led groups can offer social support and shared coping strategies.

BOTH OCD AND PTSD ARE complex disorders that require a multi-faceted treatment approach for effective management. Timely intervention is crucial for better long-term outcomes.

Late-Onset Disorders

Late-Onset Anxiety Disorders

Core Features:

- **Excessive Worry**: Generalized fears and anxieties.
- **Physical Symptoms**: Palpitations, shaking, dizziness.

Onset:

- **Middle Age or Older**: Sometimes associated with the onset of medical conditions, or the psychological stress of aging and associated life changes.

Treatment Options:

- **Anxiolytics**: Medication like benzodiazepines, though cautiously used in older adults due to side effects.
- **CBT**: Cognitive Behavioral Therapy.
- **Mindfulness Techniques**: To manage symptoms.

TREATMENT FOR LATE-onset conditions often involves a more cautious approach, considering potential comorbidities and the side effects of medications in older adults. Special attention is also given to differentiate symptoms from age-related cognitive and physiological changes.

Chapter34: Comorbidity

Co-morbidity in mental health refers to the presence of more than one mental disorder in an individual at the same time. This can complicate both diagnosis and treatment, and poses a set of unique challenges:

Diagnostic Challenges

- **Overlapping Symptoms**: Many mental health disorders share symptoms, making it difficult to differentiate between them.
- **Masking**: One disorder can mask the symptoms of another, making the less prominent disorder harder to identify.
- **Severity Variance**: Co-morbid conditions may vary in severity, making it tempting to focus on the more severe disorder and neglect the other(s).

Treatment Complexities

- **Medication Interactions**: Different disorders often require different medications, which can interact in unpredictable ways.
- **Contradicting Therapies**: The best practice treatment for one disorder might be ineffective or even detrimental when treating another disorder.
- **Resource Intensive**: Treating multiple disorders

usually requires more resources, like time and specialized care, than treating a single disorder.

Impact on Daily Life

- **Compounded Stigma**: The societal stigma associated with mental health issues can be more pronounced for those with multiple diagnoses.
- **Quality of Life**: Multiple disorders often result in a more significant impact on an individual's overall quality of life.
- **Functional Impairment**: The combined effect of multiple disorders can result in more severe functional impairments in social, occupational, or other important settings.

Therapeutic Approaches

- **Integrated Treatment Plans**: These aim to address all identified disorders rather than treating each one in isolation.
- **Multi-disciplinary Team**: Psychiatrists, psychologists, social workers, and occupational therapists may all be involved in the treatment plan.
- **Tailored Psychotherapy**: Specialized forms of psychotherapy may be employed, such as a combination of CBT for anxiety and Dialectical Behavior Therapy (DBT) for emotional regulation in the case of co-morbid anxiety and Borderline Personality Disorder.

Ethical and Clinical Considerations

- **Informed Consent**: Complexity increases when managing multiple conditions, making it crucial that patients are fully aware of all aspects of their treatment.
- **Confidentiality**: With a larger team of healthcare providers involved, maintaining patient confidentiality becomes more challenging.

UNDERSTANDING THE COMPLEXITIES of co-morbid mental health conditions is crucial for healthcare providers to deliver effective, comprehensive care. It often requires a more nuanced and integrated approach, highly customized to meet the specific needs of each individual.

Chapter 35: Alternative Diagnosis

Misdiagnoses in mental health can have serious consequences, affecting treatment plans and long-term outcomes. The process of mental health diagnosis is complex and often complicated by overlapping symptoms among different disorders. Here are some commonly misdiagnosed mental health conditions:

Bipolar Disorder

- Often misdiagnosed as Major Depressive Disorder due to the similarities in their depressive phases. People may seek treatment for depression without mentioning episodes of mania or hypomania, which are critical for a bipolar diagnosis.

ADHD (Attention-Deficit/Hyperactivity Disorder)

- Frequently mistaken for mood disorders or anxiety disorders, especially in adults who may describe their symptoms as stress or mood swings rather than attention issues.

Autism Spectrum Disorder

- May be overlooked in high-functioning individuals and misdiagnosed as ADHD or a personality disorder like Obsessive-Compulsive Disorder.

Borderline Personality Disorder

- Sometimes misdiagnosed as Bipolar Disorder due to its mood instability. Conversely, its hallmark symptom of fear of abandonment can sometimes lead to a misdiagnosis of dependent personality disorder or anxiety disorders.

Generalized Anxiety Disorder (GAD)

- Can be mistaken for depression, as the worry and physical symptoms like fatigue and poor concentration can overlap with depressive symptoms.

Dissociative Identity Disorder (DID)

- Frequently misdiagnosed as schizophrenia, bipolar disorder, or borderline personality disorder due to the complexity and variability of symptoms.

Schizophrenia

- May be misdiagnosed as Bipolar Disorder or even as a substance abuse disorder due to overlapping symptoms like delusions or hallucinations.

Somatic Symptom Disorder

- Often misdiagnosed as a medical condition, as

people with this disorder experience real physical symptoms.

Obsessive-Compulsive Disorder (OCD)

- Sometimes confused with Generalized Anxiety Disorder (GAD) or even an eating disorder due to the rituals and intrusive thoughts.

Post-Traumatic Stress Disorder (PTSD)

- May be misdiagnosed as generalized anxiety disorder or major depressive disorder if the trauma history is not adequately assessed.

IT IS ESSENTIAL TO note that a correct diagnosis often requires a comprehensive evaluation, including medical history, symptoms, and often several sessions with mental health professionals. Sometimes, co-occurring disorders make diagnosis and treatment planning even more complex. Due to the risk of misdiagnosis, second opinions and longitudinal assessments are often recommended.

Chapter 36: Substance Abuse

The relationship between substance abuse and mental health is often complex and bidirectional, meaning one can exacerbate the other and vice versa. Here are some key points to consider:

Co-occurrence and Co-morbidity

- **Self-Medication**: Individuals with mental health conditions may use substances to alleviate symptoms, although this often worsens the condition over time.
- **Increased Risk**: Substance abuse can increase the risk of developing mental health conditions and also make existing conditions worse.
- **Synergistic Effects**: The simultaneous presence of a mental health condition and substance abuse often creates a cycle that exacerbates both, making each condition more severe than it would be on its own.

Diagnostic Challenges

- **Symptom Overlap**: Both mental health conditions and substance abuse can share symptoms like mood swings, anxiety, and depression, complicating the diagnosis.
- **Temporal Sequence**: It can be difficult to determine which came first, the substance abuse or the mental

health condition, making treatment planning
complex.

Treatment Complexities

- **Integrated Treatment**: Best practices often involve treating both conditions concurrently rather than one at a time.
- **Medication Management**: Some medications used for mental health conditions can interact negatively with substances, complicating treatment.
- **Relapse Risks**: Substance abuse increases the risk of relapse for mental health conditions and vice versa.

Social and Societal Impact

- **Stigma**: Both substance abuse and mental health conditions face social stigmas that can deter individuals from seeking treatment.
- **Legal Issues**: Substance abuse can result in legal problems that may complicate the treatment of mental health conditions.

Treatment Approaches

- **Dual Diagnosis Programs**: These are specialized treatment programs designed to treat both substance abuse and co-occurring mental health conditions.
- **Cognitive Behavioral Therapy (CBT)**: This can be effective for treating both substance abuse and a

range of mental health conditions.

- **Pharmacotherapy**: Medications such as anti-depressants or antipsychotics may be used to treat the mental health aspect while medications like methadone can be used for substance abuse treatment.

BY UNDERSTANDING THE intricate relationship between substance abuse and mental health, clinicians can better tailor treatment plans to address the complex needs of individuals facing these dual challenges. Integrated and comprehensive care is often the most effective approach for these complex cases.

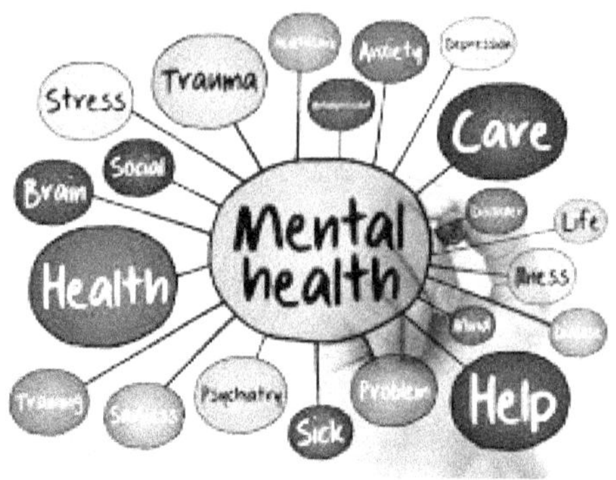

Stress
Trauma
Anxiety
Depression
Care
Social
Brain
Life
Health
Illness
Training
Psychiatry
Sick
Problem
Help
Mental health

PART FOUR: Getting Better

Chapter 37: Legal & Ethical Situation

In the United Kingdom, legal and ethical issues surrounding mental health are largely regulated by several key pieces of legislation and ethical guidelines. These legal frameworks aim to balance individual autonomy with the need to protect those at risk of harming themselves or others.

Mental Health Act 1983 (Amended 2007)

- **Involuntary Commitment**: Also known as "sectioning," this law allows medical professionals to detain individuals for their own safety or the safety of others.
- **Rights of the Detained**: The Act outlines the rights and treatment of individuals who have been involuntarily committed, including the right to appeal.
- **Tribunals**: Patients have the right to challenge their detention through Mental Health Tribunals.

Mental Capacity Act 2005

- **Best Interests**: When an individual lacks the capacity to make a decision, any action taken must be in their best interests.
- **Lasting Power of Attorney**: Allows individuals to

appoint someone to make decisions on their behalf should they lose mental capacity in the future.

Data Protection Act 2018 and Confidentiality

- **Confidentiality**: Health professionals are obligated to keep information confidential unless there's a risk to the individual's life or to public safety.
- **Information Sharing**: In complex cases involving multiple disorders or co-morbid conditions, multidisciplinary teams may need to share information, raising ethical concerns about confidentiality.

The Human Rights Act 1998

- **Article 3**: Prohibits torture and inhumane or degrading treatment, which applies to mental health treatment settings.
- **Article 8**: Respects the right to private and family life, which can come into play when considering the involuntary commitment of an individual.

Professional Guidelines

- **General Medical Council**: Provides ethical guidelines for doctors, including those related to confidentiality and informed consent.
- **British Psychological Society**: Also issues ethical guidelines that psychologists are expected to follow,

including in the assessment and treatment of mental disorders.

Ethical Issues Specific to Substance Abuse

- **Confidentiality vs Public Safety**: Especially relevant for substance abuse cases where the individual might pose a danger to the public (e.g., driving under the influence).
- **Involuntary Detoxification**: This remains a debated issue—when, if ever, it is ethical to forcibly detain someone for substance abuse treatment.

Ethical Considerations in Co-morbidity

- **Informed Consent**: In the case of co-morbid mental health and substance abuse disorders, obtaining informed consent for treatment can be more complex.
- **Balancing Treatments**: Ethical issues can arise when determining which condition to treat first or how to adapt treatment modalities to address both conditions safely.

THE LEGAL AND ETHICAL frameworks in the UK aim to provide a comprehensive, human-rights-focused approach to mental health care. Nonetheless, these systems are continuously evolving, particularly as societal attitudes towards mental health continue to change.

Scotland has its own legal framework for dealing with mental health issues, which often complements UK-wide legislation but also has distinct differences. One key piece of legislation is the Mental Health (Care and Treatment) (Scotland) Act 2003.

Mental Health (Care and Treatment) (Scotland) Act 2003

- **Emergency Detention**: Allows for an individual to be detained for up to 72 hours for assessment, usually requiring the consent of a Mental Health Officer (MHO).
- **Short-term Detention**: Allows for detention up to 28 days, requiring certification by a medical practitioner and consent from an MHO.
- **Compulsory Treatment Order (CTO)**: This can last for six months initially, then be renewed for six months and subsequently for 12 months at a time.
- **Safeguards**: Patients have the right to appeal, and there are provisions for independent advocacy.

Adults with Incapacity (Scotland) Act 2000

- **Financial and Welfare Guardianship**: This allows a guardian to be appointed to manage the welfare and/ or finances of an adult who lacks capacity.

- **Power of Attorney**: Like the Mental Capacity Act 2005 in the rest of the UK, this act also allows for individuals to appoint someone to make decisions on their behalf if they become incapacitated.

Scottish Mental Welfare Commission

- This body oversees the welfare of individuals with mental illness, learning disabilities, and related conditions. It provides guidance, monitors the use of legislation, and can investigate cases.

Confidentiality and Data Sharing

- Scotland has its own guidelines for medical confidentiality and data protection in healthcare settings, although these are generally aligned with UK-wide standards.

Alcohol and Drug Treatment

- Scotland has specific laws and programs aimed at reducing substance abuse, which are particularly relevant for co-morbid mental health conditions.

THE SCOTTISH LEGAL system places a significant emphasis on human rights, patients' rights, and ethical considerations, much like the broader UK system. However, it operates under its own legal framework, and those practicing in Scotland need to be aware of these unique aspects.

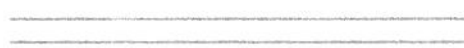

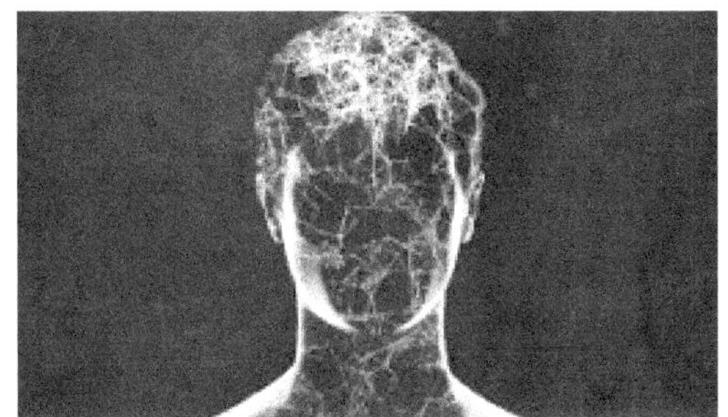

Chapter 38: Medication / Drugs

Here are some of the most common prescribed medications. Some brand names may be different outside of the U.K.

A - Antipsychotics

- **Aripiprazole (Abilify)**: Used to treat schizophrenia, bipolar disorder, and as an adjunct in depressive disorders. It balances certain neurotransmitters in the brain.

B - Benzodiazepines

- **Lorazepam (Ativan)**: Primarily used for anxiety disorders and insomnia. It works by slowing down brain activity.
- **Diazepam (Valium)**: Used for anxiety, muscle spasms, and seizures. It calms the nervous system.

C - Cyclic Antidepressants

- **Amitriptyline**: Used for depression, neuropathic pain, and migraine prevention. It increases serotonin and norepinephrine levels.
- **Nortriptyline (Allegron)**: Mainly for depression. It also alters mood by affecting neurotransmitters.

D - Dopamine Agonists

- **Pramipexole (Mirapexin)**: Primarily for Parkinson's disease, but also used off-label for mood disorders. It mimics the effects of dopamine.

E - SSRIs (Selective Serotonin Reuptake Inhibitors)

- **Escitalopram (Cipralex)**: For depression and generalized anxiety disorder. It increases serotonin levels in the brain.
- **Fluoxetine (Prozac)**: For depression, OCD, and panic disorder. It also affects serotonin levels.

F - SNRIs (Serotonin-Norepinephrine Reuptake Inhibitors)

- **Venlafaxine (Efexor)**: For depression, anxiety, and panic disorders. It affects both serotonin and norepinephrine.
- **Duloxetine (Cymbalta, Yentreve)**: For depression, generalized anxiety, and neuropathic pain. It also influences serotonin and norepinephrine.

G - GABA Reuptake Inhibitors

- **Tiagabine (Gabitril)**: Used for epilepsy and sometimes for anxiety off-label. It inhibits the reuptake of GABA.

H - Histamine Receptor Antagonists

- **Hydroxyzine (Atarax, Ucerax)**: For short-term anxiety and tension. It blocks histamine receptors.

I - Iproniazid

- An older MAOI used for treatment-resistant depression. It inhibits the enzyme that breaks down neurotransmitters like serotonin and dopamine.

L - Lithium

- A mood stabilizer for bipolar disorder and treatment-resistant depression. It's not entirely clear how it works but is thought to affect various neurotransmitters and hormones.

M - MAOIs (Monoamine Oxidase Inhibitors)

- **Phenelzine (Nardil)**: For treatment-resistant depression. It inhibits an enzyme that breaks down mood-enhancing neurotransmitters.

N - NMDA Receptor Antagonists

- **Memantine (Ebixa, Maruxa)**: Primarily for Alzheimer's but used off-label for mood disorders. It modulates glutamatergic neurotransmission.

O - Opioids

- **Buprenorphine (Subutex)**: Sometimes used off-label for severe, treatment-resistant depression. It partially activates opioid receptors.

P - Pregabalin (Lyrica)

- For neuropathic pain and generalized anxiety disorder. It modulates calcium channel activity.

Q - Quetiapine (Seroquel)

- For schizophrenia, bipolar, and adjunctive treatment of depression. It affects multiple neurotransmitters.

R - Reboxetine (Edronax)

- A norepinephrine reuptake inhibitor for depression. It enhances norepinephrine levels in the brain.

S - Stimulants

- **Methylphenidate (Ritalin, Concerta)**: For ADHD. It affects dopamine and norepinephrine levels.
- **Dexamfetamine**: Used for ADHD. Similar to Adderall, it increases levels of dopamine and norepinephrine.

T - Tetracyclic Antidepressants

- **Maprotiline**: For depression and anxiety disorders. It affects norepinephrine and, to a lesser extent, serotonin.

V - Valproate (Epilim)

- For bipolar disorder and epilepsy. It stabilizes electrical activity in the brain.

Z - Zolpidem (Stilnoct)

- For short-term treatment of insomnia. It depresses the central nervous system.

PLEASE CONSULT WITH healthcare providers for an accurate diagnosis and appropriate medication. This list is not exhaustive and should be tailored to individual needs.

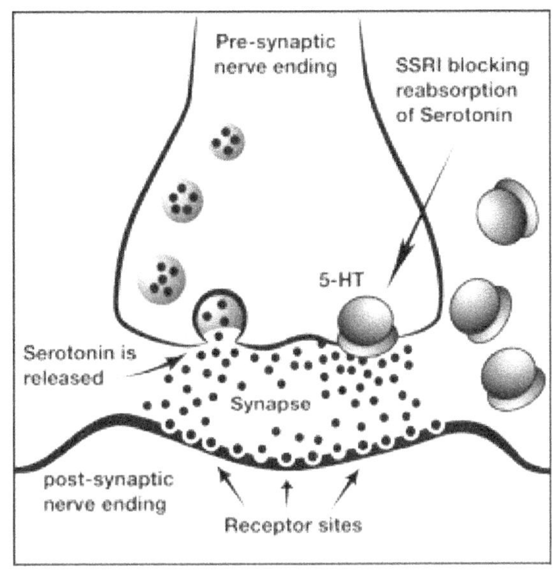

Pre-synaptic
nerve ending
SSRI blocking
reabsorption
of Serotonin
5-HT
Serotonin is
released
Synapse
post-synaptic
nerve ending
Receptor sites

Chapter 39: Alternative / Complimentary Treatments

There are various alternative or complementary therapies available for mental health treatment. These approaches are often used alongside conventional medical treatments, but some people also use them independently. Here are some of the alternative therapies commonly used:

Mindfulness and Meditation

THESE PRACTICES ORIGINATE from ancient Buddhist and Hindu traditions but have been widely adopted in Western psychology due to their proven effectiveness in reducing symptoms of stress, anxiety, and depression. Mindfulness-based cognitive therapy (MBCT) and mindfulness-based stress reduction (MBSR) are structured programs that incorporate mindfulness to improve mental well-being.

How It Works:

MINDFULNESS INVOLVES moment-to-moment awareness and acceptance of one's thoughts and feelings. This increased awareness can help individuals recognize problematic thought patterns and develop more adaptive reactions to stress.

Acupuncture

THIS ANCIENT CHINESE practice aims to balance the body's energy channels, known as meridians, by inserting thin needles into specific points on the body.

How It Works:

THE INSERTION POINTS correspond to various body systems, and the process is thought to stimulate the nervous system. This can release endorphins, providing a natural painkiller effect and potentially elevating mood.

Yoga

YOGA IS AN ANCIENT practice originating in India that combines physical postures, breath control, and meditation.

How It Works:

VARIOUS STYLES OF YOGA, such as Hatha, Vinyasa, or Kundalini, focus on different aspects of the practice, but all aim to balance the mind, body, and spirit. Specific poses and breathing techniques can help focus the mind and reduce anxiety and stress.

Herbal Medicine

HERBAL REMEDIES HAVE been used for centuries to treat a range of ailments, including mental health conditions.

How It Works:

DIFFERENT HERBS LIKE St. John's Wort for mild depression, Valerian root for anxiety, and Kava for stress have varying degrees of effectiveness, supported by different levels of scientific evidence. It's crucial to consult with a healthcare provider because some herbs can interact with medications or worsen certain medical conditions.

Nutritional Supplements

VARIOUS SUPPLEMENTS aim to support mental health by providing essential nutrients that may be lacking in the diet.

How It Works:

OMEGA-3 FATTY ACIDS, often found in fish oil supplements, have shown promise in treating symptoms of depression and anxiety. Amino acids like L-Theanine can also help with stress and focus.

Biofeedback

BIOFEEDBACK USES ELECTRONIC monitoring to convey information about physiological processes.

How It Works:

BY LEARNING HOW TO interpret these physiological cues—like heart rate, skin temperature, and muscle tension—individuals can gain better control over their stress and anxiety responses. This method is particularly useful for conditions like anxiety and ADHD.

Art and Music Therapy

THESE THERAPIES ALLOW for emotional expression through creative outlets, whether it's painting, drawing, or making music.

How It Works:

CREATING ART OR MUSIC can be a non-threatening way to explore emotions and experiences. These therapies are often used in settings that treat trauma, anxiety, and depression.

It's worth noting that while these alternative therapies can be effective, they should not replace traditional medical treatments, especially for severe mental health conditions. Always consult with a healthcare provider for a comprehensive treatment plan tailored to your individual needs.

Chapter 40: Life Expectancy

Schizophrenia

Studies suggest that men with schizophrenia may have a life expectancy reduced by up to 25 years, whereas for women it might be reduced by up to 20 years. The reduction in life expectancy is often due to increased physical health issues and a higher rate of suicide.

Bipolar Disorder

MEN WITH BIPOLAR DISORDER can see their life expectancy reduced by 13 to 20 years. For women, it could be around 12 to 15 years less. The difference is attributed to an increased likelihood of cardiovascular disease among men.

Major Depressive Disorder

WOMEN WITH MAJOR DEPRESSIVE disorder might have a life expectancy reduced by about 10 to 12 years, whereas men could have theirs reduced by approximately 12 to 14 years. Men are generally less likely to be diagnosed but often experience more severe symptoms and a higher rate of suicide.

Anxiety Disorders

THOUGH THE IMPACT ON life expectancy is less severe than other conditions, men might experience a reduction of 2 to 5 years, and women about 1 to 3 years. Anxiety disorders often co-occur with other physical or mental conditions, complicating these estimates.

Personality Disorders

MEN WITH CERTAIN PERSONALITY disorders (e.g., borderline, antisocial) may see their life expectancy reduced significantly, primarily due to a higher likelihood of engaging in risky behaviors or dying by suicide. For women, the data is less clear but still suggests a reduced life expectancy.

Eating Disorders

WOMEN WITH ANOREXIA nervosa can have a life expectancy reduced by 20 to 25 years. Men, who are less frequently diagnosed, can experience even more severe reductions when they do have the disorder.

UK-Specific Data

UK-SPECIFIC DATA OFTEN aligns with these general findings. The NHS and publications like The Lancet often provide statistical data on these subjects.

It's essential to note that these are statistical figures and not destiny. Many people with these conditions live long, fulfilling lives, particularly with effective treatment and support.

For the most up-to-date and comprehensive information, it would be best to consult academic journals, healthcare organizations, and statistical databases.

Sources

IT'S IMPORTANT TO CONSULT academic journals, public health organizations, and other reliable sources for the most up-to-date information.

Finally, it's crucial to note that effective treatment and lifestyle changes can often significantly improve life expectancy and quality of life for people with these conditions.

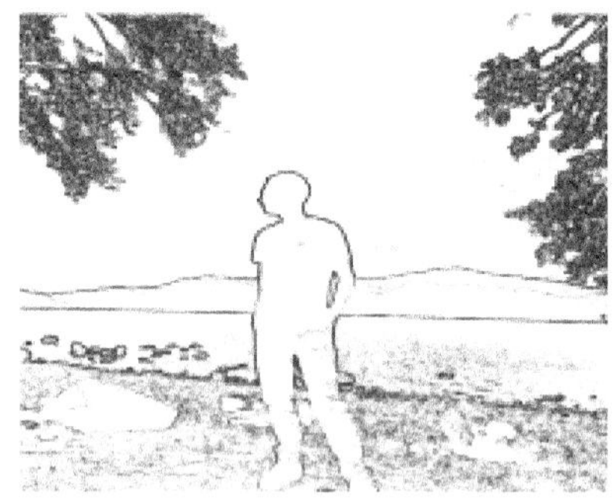

Chapter 41: Resources

Public Health Services

1. **NHS Mental Health Services**: These services range from psychological therapies (also known as talking therapies) to specialized psychiatric care. Patients usually need a referral from a General Practitioner (GP) to access these services.
     - **Community Mental Health Teams (CMHTs)**: Offer support for a wide range of mental health issues and act as the primary point of care for continued treatment.

1. **Improving Access to Psychological Therapies (IAPT)**: This NHS programme offers a range of treatments, including cognitive behavioral therapy (CBT), for individuals with anxiety and depression.
2. **Child and Adolescent Mental Health Services (CAMHS)**: These are specialized services offering assessment and treatment to children and young people up to the age of 18 who have emotional, behavioral, or mental health difficulties.

General UK Helplines

1. **Samaritans**: 116 123 (Open 24/7)
2. **Mind Infoline**: 0300 123 3393 (Various hours)

3. **CALM (Campaign Against Living Miserably)**: 0800 58 58 58 (5 pm to midnight daily)
4. **SANE**: 0300 304 7000 (4:30 pm to 10:30 pm daily)
5. **Papyrus**: 0800 068 4141 (9 am to midnight daily)
6. **Childline**: 0800 1111 (Open 24/7)
7. **Silver Line**: 0800 4 70 80 90 (Open 24/7)
8. **No Panic**: 0844 967 4848 (10 am to 10 pm daily)
9. **Rethink Mental Illness**: 0300 5000 927 (Various hours)
10. **YoungMinds**: 0808 802 5544 (9:30 am to 4 pm, Monday to Friday)
11. **Anxiety UK**: 03444 775 774 (Mon-Fri 9:30 am - 10 pm, weekends 10 am - 8 pm)
12. **FRANK**: 0300 123 6600 (Open 24/7)
13. **Women's Aid**: 0808 2000 247 (Open 24/7)
14. **LGBT+ Helpline (Switchboard)**: 0300 330 0630 (10 am to 10 pm daily)

Scotland-Specific Helplines

1. **Breathing Space**: 0800 83 85 87 (6 pm to 2 am weekdays, 24 hours on weekends)
2. **SAMH (Scottish Association for Mental Health)**: 0141 530 1000 (Various hours)
3. **Edinburgh Crisis Centre**: 0808 801 0414 (Open 24/7)
4. **NHS 24**: 111 (Open 24/7)
5. **Rape Crisis Scotland**: 08088 01 03 02 (6 pm to midnight)
6. **Men Matter Scotland**: No specific helpline, but they

offer online support and resources on their website.

A lways double-check the helpline's website or call them for the most current and accurate information.

Conclusion

As we draw the curtain on this exhaustive journey through the A to Z of mental health terms, conditions, and resources, it's essential to remember that the landscape of mental health is both broad and complex. Mental health doesn't discriminate; it can affect anyone, regardless of age, gender, socio-economic background, or geographical location.

Our aim has been not merely to inform but to empower you—the reader—with the knowledge needed to navigate the intricate labyrinth of mental health. Whether you are an individual coping with a mental health condition, a concerned family member, or a healthcare provider, understanding the terminology and available resources can be a transformative first step. We've delved into the details of various conditions, from Cluster A, B, and C personality disorders to other non-categorical conditions. We've discussed treatment options, both pharmaceutical and therapeutic, and have even shed light on the legal landscape in the UK, with special mention of Scottish-specific considerations.

We must also acknowledge the persistent societal stigma attached to mental health. While progress has been made, the path ahead remains steep. It's vital to challenge and change our collective perceptions, to humanise rather than label, and to embrace vulnerability as a facet of the human experience. The resources and helplines listed throughout this book serve as lifelines, but they also stand as testament to the work done by countless individuals and organisations who are challenging the stigma, one conversation at a time.

To those of you who battle your own minds every day, know that you are not alone. This book is a testament to human resilience and an invitation to collective responsibility. The conversation doesn't end on these pages—it begins. Let's carry it into our homes, workplaces, and communities. Let's be vigilant and active, listening and speaking, until the dialogue surrounding mental health is as common and accepted as any other facet of human health.

We're all a part of this tapestry, each thread as crucial as the next. Whether you're seeking help, offering it, or advocating for it, your role is indispensable. The key to better mental health is both individual and collective action, and this book hopes to be a stepping stone in that crucial endeavour.

Thank you for joining us on this educational journey. May the knowledge you've gained here equip you to face life's challenges with greater understanding, compassion, and resilience.

Your journey in understanding and navigating the complex sphere of mental health has only just begun, and we are hopeful that this book has provided you with the tools you need to take the next steps. Take care.

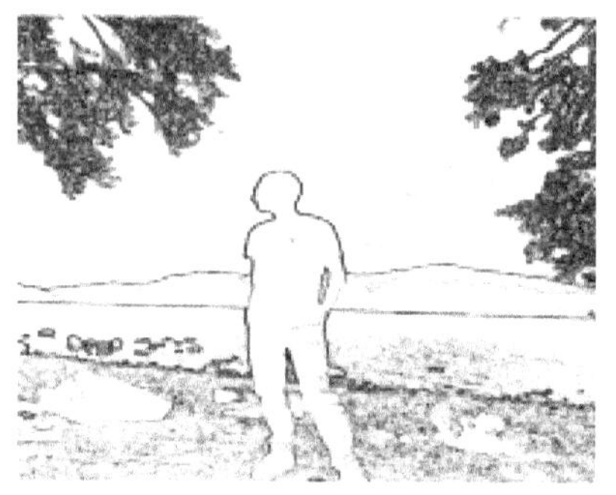